Military Medicine and the Making of Race

This book demonstrates how Britain's black soldiers helped shape attitudes towards race throughout the nineteenth century. Part of the British military establishment for 132 years, the West India Regiments generated vast records, with details about every one of their more than 100,000 recruits, making them the best-documented group of black men in the Atlantic World. Tim Lockley shows how, in the late eighteenth century, surgeons established in medical literature that white and black bodies were radically different, forging a notion of the 'superhuman' black soldier able to undertake physical challenges far beyond the abilities of white soldiers. By the late 1830s, however, military statisticians would contest these ideas and instead highlight the vulnerabilities of black soldiers. The popularity and pervasiveness of these publications spread far beyond British military or medical circles and had a significant international impact, particularly in the United States, both reflecting and reinforcing changing notions about blackness.

Tim Lockley is Professor of North American history at the University of Warwick and the author of *Lines in the Sand: Race and Class in Lowcountry Georgia, 1750–1860* (2001), *Welfare and Charity in the Antebellum South* (2007) and *Maroon Communities in South Carolina* (2009).

Military Medicine and the Making of Race

Life and Death in the West India Regiments, 1795–1874

Tim Lockley

University of Warwick

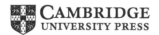

CAMBRIDGE
UNIVERSITY PRESS

University Printing House, Cambridge CB2 8BS, United Kingdom

One Liberty Plaza, 20th Floor, New York, NY 10006, USA

477 Williamstown Road, Port Melbourne, VIC 3207, Australia

314-321, 3rd Floor, Plot 3, Splendor Forum, Jasola District Centre, New Delhi - 110025, India

103 Penang Road, #05-06/07, Visioncrest Commercial, Singapore 238467

Cambridge University Press is part of the University of Cambridge.

It furthers the University's mission by disseminating knowledge in the pursuit of education, learning and research at the highest international levels of excellence.

www.cambridge.org
Information on this title: www.cambridge.org/9781108797139
DOI: 10.1017/9781108862417

First published 2020
First paperback edition 2022

A catalogue record for this publication is available from the British Library

Library of Congress Cataloging in Publication data
Names: Lockley, Timothy James, 1971- author.
Title: Military medicine and the making of race : life and death in the West India regiments, 1795-1874 / Tim Lockley, University of Warwick.
Description: New York, NY : Cambridge University Press, 2020. | Includes bibliographical references and index.
Identifiers: LCCN 2019043911 | ISBN 9781108495622 (hardback) | ISBN 9781108495622 (ebook)
Subjects: LCSH: Blacks--Race identity--West Indies, British--History--18th century. | Blacks--Race identity--West Indies, British--History--19th century. | Great Britain. Army--Colonial forces--West Indies, British--History. | Soldiers, Black--West Indies, British--History. | Race relations--West Indies, British. | Medicine, Military--West Indies, British--History--19th century.
Classification: LCC HT1581 .L63 2020 | DDC 305.896/0729--dc23
LC record available at https://lccn.loc.gov/2019043911

ISBN 978-1-108-49562-2 Hardback
ISBN 978-1-108-79713-9 Paperback

For Emma, who was not even born
when I wrote my last book

Contents

Figures and Tables

Figures

Tables

Acknowledgements

Although this book builds on themes that I have previously worked on, particularly related to the history of medicine, studying the West India Regiments has introduced me to military history for the first time as well as the histories of the Caribbean and West Africa. Undoubtedly the spark was a conversation with my colleague at Warwick, David Lambert, who suggested we put together a team of people to work on the West India Regiments. With the assistance of my former research student David Doddington (now an established academic in his own right) and some seed funding from our university, we wrote an ambitious proposal to the Arts and Humanities Research Council (AHRC) for a four-year project grant. Getting funding is something of a lottery as many very good proposals are not funded, but we were awarded a little over £500,000. My thanks to the anonymous AHRC reviewers and panellists who believed in our vision. The project team of myself, David Lambert, Elizabeth Cooper from the British Library, and two doctoral students, Melissa Bennett and Rosalyn Narayan, were ably assisted by our advisory board of Ria Bartlett, Gad Heuman, David Killingray and Kay Dian Kriz. Throughout the four years we collaborated extremely effectively. Each team member had their own part of the project, of course, but we shared archival tips and resources and we all contributed to our two major engagement activities, an exhibition at the Museum of London Docklands and an online learning resource hosted by the British Library. Huge thanks to the staff at both institutions for helping us deliver these crucial parts of our project. We held a project conference 'Armed People of African Descent: Africa and the Americas, 1750–1900' at Warwick in May 2017 and produced a special issue of *Slavery and Abolition* arising from it in September 2018. Thanks to Gad Heuman for helping us do this.

Most of the archival research was undertaken at the National Archives in Kew, with additional visits to the British Library, the Wellcome Library, the Library of Congress and the South Caroliniana Library. Thanks to all the staff from those institutions for their help and advice.

I presented some of the ideas in this book at a number of conferences, including BrANCH, EEASA, BGEAH and the AHA, and spoke to seminars at a number of universities. I appreciate all of those who made thoughtful and insightful comments. The anonymous readers for Cambridge University Press were also incredibly helpful, and the book is certainly better for their advice.

Lastly, the tolerance and encouragement of Jo, Alice, Ed and Emma was absolutely vital in the completion of this project. Research trips abroad certainly gave Jo extra work and stress, and the kids all had to adjust as their usual routines were changed. Alice did some great ferrying around of her siblings, while Ed had to get up early (much too early he would say) to walk the dogs. Thanks also to my mum who came and helped out on several occasions.

Any book is something of a collaborative effort. My name might be on the cover but, as these acknowledgements prove, lots of people have been involved behind the scenes. Heartfelt thanks to all of them.

Introduction

This book is about race. Specifically, it is about the development of racial thought from the end of the eighteenth century through to the second half of the nineteenth century. It starts with one war – Britain's epic struggle with France between 1793 and 1815 – and ends with another – the Anglo-Asante War of 1873–4, neatly sidestepping the American Civil War in between. It is apt that warfare bookends this study since the main focus of the book are the West India Regiments (WIRs), British army units composed largely of men of African descent. This book uses the WIRs as a lens to focus in on changing racial attitudes in the anglophone Atlantic.

Racial Thought

Race is a slippery concept. As a means of categorising peoples it has only a tangential relationship with biology.[1] It is far too subjective, and often personal, for that. As individuals we each perceive race differently, primarily via sight but with the other senses contributing as well, constructing a racial identity for ourselves and for others that may not concord with those of other people.[2] Someone whom I perceive to be white, for instance, might not be perceived by others as white, or indeed think of themselves as white. If race is confusing now, it was an even more plastic concept for most of the seventeenth and eighteenth centuries, 'being determined by lifestyles, diet and, above all, by climate'.[3]

---

[1] Barbara J. Fields, 'Ideology and race in American history', in J. Morgan Kousset and James M. McPherson (eds.), *Region, Race and Reconstruction: Essays in Honor of C. Vann Woodward* (New York: Oxford University Press, 1982), 143–77.

[2] For the importance of all the senses in racial categorisation, see Mark M. Smith, *How Race Is Made: Slavery, Segregation and the Senses* (Chapel Hill: University of North Carolina Press, 2006).

[3] Mark Harrison, *Climates and Constitutions: Health, Race, Environment and British Imperialism in India, 1600–1850* (Oxford: Oxford University Press, 1999), 11; Sharon Block, *Colonial Complexions: Race and Bodies in Eighteenth-Century America* (Philadelphia: University of Pennsylvania Press, 2018), 33.

Skin colour, usually given primacy as a means of racial categorisation today, was just one means of classifying and describing bodies. As Edward Beasley has put it, before the late eighteenth century there was 'no idea of race as we have come to know it – no widely shared theory of biologically determined, physical, intellectual, and moral differences between different human groups'.[4] English trader Bartholomew Stibbs, visiting the Gambia River in 1723, remarked, without apparent irony, that the local inhabitants were 'as Black as Coal; tho' here, thro' Custom, (being Christians) they account themselves White Men'.[5] This lack of intellectual coherence left gaps that individual non-whites were able to exploit, asserting rights to freedom, land and even suffrage for a period, that were normally reserved for whites.[6]

But fluidity in racial thought did not translate to better treatment of non-whites. As Europeans explored the world, they were supremely confident of their own moral, religious and technological superiority over all non-European people, whether Amerindian, Asian or African.[7] After all, it was Europeans who instituted a system of plantation slavery in the Americas that involved the involuntary labour of millions of Amerindians and Africans, and the deaths of a high percentage of them.[8] Yet historians have noted a clear evolution in racial thinking during the later eighteenth and first half of the nineteenth centuries. Skin colour became the predominant racial marker, and demarcations between whites and non-whites became clearer throughout the Atlantic World, both legally and culturally. Whites came to what Roxann Wheeler has described as a form of 'cultural consensus' about their rightful dominance over all others.[9] Whites ruled simply because they

---

[4] Edward Beasley, *The Victorian Reinvention of Race* (New York: Routledge, 2010), 1.

[5] 'Journal of a voyage up the Gambia', printed in Francis Moore, *Travels into the Inland Parts of Africa* (London: Edward Cave, 1738), 243.

[6] T. H. Breen and Stephen Innes, *'Myne Owne Ground': Race and Freedom on Virginia's Eastern Shore, 1640–1676*, 2nd ed. (Oxford: Oxford University Press, 2005), 10–17.

[7] The best short summary of English attitudes towards non-whites in the early modern period remains Winthrop Jordan, *White over Black: American Attitudes towards the Negro* (Chapel Hill: University of North Carolina Press, 1968), 3–43. For the link between Iberian and Anglo-American attitudes, see James H. Sweet, 'The Iberian roots of American racist thought', *William and Mary Quarterly* 54 (1997), 143–66.

[8] Between 1640 and 1700, 264,000 slaves were imported into the British West Indies, but in 1700 the enslaved population was only 100,000. Richard S. Dunn, *Sugar and Slaves: the Rise of the Planter Class in the English West Indies, 1624–1713* (Chapel Hill: University of North Carolina Press, 1972), 314.

[9] Roxann Wheeler, *The Complexion of Race: Categories of Difference in Eighteenth-Century British Culture* (Philadelphia: University of Pennsylvania Press, 2000), 240.

were white, and blacks toiled because they were black. Racial categories as a result became fixed and unalterable and were the most important way colonisers defined themselves in opposition to the colonised. Heathens might become Christian, the uncivilised might become educated, but black people could not be transformed into white people. Race had always been important, particularly so in the Americas, but, as one writer put it, by 1850 'race is everything', with political, economic and social ascendancy granted to whites and denied to others.[10]

A common explanation for this transformation of racial attitudes points to slavery as the culprit.[11] The most typical encounter between white people and those of African descent involved enslavement in the Americas, with the attitudes of those coming from Europe being continuously moulded by the denigration, mistreatment and objectification of black bodies.[12] When voices began to be heard challenging enslavement from the 1770s and 1780s on, new and powerful justifications for the system were required, spelling out the clear differences between black and white people. These rationales claimed, among other things, that black people were intellectually incapable of becoming truly civilised and needed white protection, guidance and supervision.[13] Despite slavery ending in the US northern states, and subsequently in the British Caribbean, racial attitudes in anglophone societies continued this hardening trend. Indeed, as Britain's imperial tentacles began to reach every corner of the globe, involving the subjection of an immense variety of different peoples, ideas concerning 'separate, stable, physically distinct, and physically inheritable races' firmly established themselves as the intellectual mainstream.[14]

But an alternative and complementary story can be told about evolving racial attitudes, one that does not revolve around enslavement. Slavery, in some senses, overly dominates of our understanding of how black people were perceived in the late eighteenth and early nineteenth

---

[10] Robert Knox, *Races of Men: a Fragment* (Philadelphia: Lea and Blanchard, 1850), 7.

[11] Jordan, *White over Black*, 429–541; Seymour Drescher, 'The ending of the slave trade and the evolution of European scientific racism', *Social Science History* 14 (1990), 415–50.

[12] Winthrop Jordan, *The White Man's Burden: Historical Origins of Racism in the United States* (New York: Oxford University Press, 1974), 26–54.

[13] See Jeffrey Robert Young (ed.), *Proslavery and Sectional Thought in the Early South, 1740–1829* (Columbia: University of South Carolina Press, 2006). Examples of those speaking out include John Wesley, *Thoughts upon Slavery* (London: R. Haws, 1774); Anthony Benezet, *The Case of Our Fellow Creatures, the Oppressed Africans* (London: James Phillips, 1784); Olaudah Equiano, *The Interesting Life of Olaudah Equiano or Gustavus Vassa, the African* (London: for the author, 1789).

[14] Beasley, *The Victorian Reinvention of Race*, 1.

centuries. Many of those writing about black people were really writing about enslaved people and concerned with denigrating or supporting the institution of slavery and not with blackness per se, though those two things were obviously intertwined to a significant degree. Free black populations existed throughout the Atlantic World, often eking out marginal existences in port towns, but few whites paid them much attention.[15] They appear in a diverse set of records generated by church vestrymen, tax collectors, census enumerators and court clerks, but rarely, if ever, systematically over a lengthy period. No one had the time or the inclination to study free black populations closely in order to establish a concept of blackness outwith the paradigm of slavery. This is where the WIRs fit into this story because they provide historians with a detailed and sustained look at a single group of black men where slavery is, for the most part, not a relevant factor.

Black Soldiers

Black soldiers were not unique to the British army, nor were they a sudden creation of the 1790s.[16] European powers had recruited black soldiers for service in the eighteenth-century Caribbean on several occasions, and in St Domingue, in a desperate last-ditch attempt to retain control, France had both ended slavery and accepted tens of thousands of former slaves into its service.[17] The WIRs stand out from

[15] See, for example, Stewart King, *Blue Coat or Powdered Wig: Free People of Color in Pre-revolutionary Saint Domingue* (Athens: University of Georgia Press, 2001); Ira Berlin, *Slaves without Masters: the Free Negro in the Antebellum South* (New York: Pantheon Books, 1974); Gad J. Heuman, *Between Black and White: Race, Politics, and the Free Coloreds in Jamaica, 1792–1865* (Westport: Greenwood Press, 1981); Christopher Phillips, *Freedom's Port: the African American Community of Baltimore, 1790–1860* (Urbana: University of Illinois Press, 1997).

[16] See, for example, Jane Landers, 'Transforming bondsmen into vassals: arming slaves in colonial Spanish America'; Hendrick Kraay, 'Arming slaves in Brazil from the seventeenth to nineteenth century'; Philip D. Morgan and Andrew O. Shaughnessy, 'Arming slaves in the American revolution'; and David Geggus, 'The arming of slaves in the Haitian revolution', all in Christopher Leslie Brown and Philip D. Morgan (eds.), *Arming Slaves from Classical Times to the Modern Age* (New Haven: Yale University Press, 2006). Peter M. Voelz, *Slave and Soldier: the Military Impact of Blacks in the Colonial Americas* (London: Garland, 1993). On black soldiers in the British army, see also Samson C. Ukpabi, 'Military recruitment and social mobility in nineteenth-century British West Africa', *Journal of African Studies* 2 (1975), 87–107; Glenford D. Howe, *Race, War and Nationalism: a Social History of West Indians in the First World War* (Oxford: James Currey, 2002); Richard Smith, *Jamaican Volunteers in the First World War: Race, Masculinity and the Development of National Consciousness* (Manchester: Manchester University Press, 2004).

[17] See David Geggus, 'The arming of slaves in the Haitian revolution' and Laurent Dubois, 'Citizen soldiers: emancipation and military service in the revolutionary French Caribbean', in Brown and Morgan, *Arming Slaves*.

these other examples of black soldiers for the simple reason that, once established in 1795, they existed in one form or another until 1927. For 132 years the regiments were a fully fledged part of the British military establishment, not a temporary corps of colonials or an informal militia, meaning they were officered just as white regiments were, and, crucially, that they generated the same bureaucracy. In addition to a normal complement of majors, captains, lieutenants and ensigns, each WIR was assigned an adjutant (responsible for overall administration), a quartermaster (overseeing supplies), a paymaster (ensuring all men were paid properly), a surgeon and an assistant surgeon (with responsibility for sanitation and healthcare). These men generated paperwork – vast quantities of it. Each wrote letters and reports to the two command headquarters in the Caribbean, in Jamaica (covering Honduras, Jamaica and the Bahamas) and in Barbados (covering the Windward and Leeward Islands, as well as Guyana), and also completed routine reports to the War Office in London. Regiments were required to report on troop strengths on a monthly basis, including the numbers who were sick and had died since the previous report, as well as those who had been recruited, transferred or invalided from service. Moreover, each regiment was inspected on a bi-annual basis by a senior commander, who examined internal management and discipline to assess whether the regiment was fit for duty. In addition, the regiment generated internal records such as pay books, regimental court martial information and muster or succession books that detailed the name of every recruit, physical information (age, height, hair and eye colour), where they were born, when and where they joined the regiment, promotions or reductions and the date and reason they left the regiment (transfer, death or retirement due to ill health or old age).

Aside from the regiments themselves, the usual operations of the British Empire and its army also generated plentiful records pertaining to the WIRs. Military commanders kept in regular touch with government ministers in Whitehall, informing them of ongoing troop movements and active campaigns, as well as pointing out operational constraints. Colonial governments were just as active, compiling huge amounts of internal information including records of legislative debates and laws passed, colonial censuses, shipping and customs data, and letters. Much of this was sent to the Colonial Office in London. The WIRs feature in many of these records, particularly when they were engaged in active operations. As the first regiments in the army containing men of African descent, the WIRs were also objects of curiosity, featuring in visitors' accounts of the West Indies, in letters written by residents to relatives elsewhere and in both local and British newspapers. Put simply, the importance of the WIRs for the study of the evolution of racial thought in the nineteenth century lies in the fact that they are the best-documented group of black men in the Atlantic World. Each regiment contained at least 500 men, and some grew to more than a thousand. In 1802 there were twelve regiments of about 500 men each, or roughly 6,000 men in total, and at the end of the century there were still more than 2,500 men serving in the West Indies and Africa.[18] During the course of the nineteenth century, the cumulative total number of men who passed through the WIRs must exceed 100,000. Even the most complete sets of plantation records are nothing like as comprehensive and, of course, cover far fewer people, though they do add vastly to our knowledge of black women who are largely absent from the records of the WIRs.[19] The nearest comparable set of data is that collected about the black soldiers fighting for the Union army during the American Civil War. There were far more of them than ever served in the WIRs but, crucially, the data only covers a very short period.[20]

Although the WIRs, by the simple virtue of being on the regular army establishment, generated vast amounts of records, not all of the data has survived to the present day. Survival depended on a number of factors, including assiduous record keeping in the first place and remembering to transfer papers along with the regiment. The WIRs were regularly rotated around the various Caribbean islands, often serving in small detachments, and from the 1820s onwards they periodically spent time in Africa. All of the earliest records of the 2WIR were lost in 1825, after being left behind in Sierra Leone when the regiment embarked for the West Indies, while those of 1WIR 'were lost in the expedition to and from New Orleans' in 1815.[21] When regiments were disbanded the records were supposed to be deposited in London, but it is clear that many were not. Moist tropical climates are not particularly conducive to record survival, and natural disasters such as hurricanes also probably took their toll. It is also clear that a

---

[18] In March 1801 the monthly return for the Windward and Leeward Islands command listed 4,640 soldiers in ten West India Regiments. The 5th and 6th WIRs are missing from these returns as they were serving in the Jamaican command. WO17/2492. *Army Medical Department Report for the Year 1898* (London: HMSO 1900), 114, 123.

[19] Some wives and children of WIR men were attached to the regiment and were mentioned in regimental returns. The women seemed to have undertaken domestic chores such as cooking for their husbands.

[20] About 180,000 black soldiers served in the Union army; see John David Smith (ed.), *Black Soldiers in Blue: African American Troops in the Civil War Era* (Chapel Hill: University of North Carolina Press, 2002).

[21] J. E. Caulfeild, *One Hundred Years' History of the 2nd Batt. West India Regiment* (London: Forster Groom, 1899), 54. *St George's Chronicle and Grenada Gazette*, 25 March 1837.

lot of records that made it back to London have subsequently been lost or destroyed. Regular reports from regimental surgeons after 1817, for instance, clearly existed in the late 1830s as they were used for statistical analysis, but few exist now. Regimental documents, including letters written to and from WIR commanders, were used for two regimental histories published towards the end of the nineteenth century, but following the disbandment of the regiment in 1927 these documents have also subsequently been lost.[22] Despite what might be termed normal record loss over the course of two centuries, vast quantities of documents remain. Many of the biannual inspection reports survive, as do some of the muster and succession books, all of the earliest pay books and most of the correspondence between commanders in chief and the War Office and between island governors and the Colonial Office. As a result, it is possible to know more about these men, how they were treated and what others thought of them, than it is for any other group of men of African descent in the nineteenth century. Generally missing, of course, are first-hand accounts written by the men themselves. We will never have a real sense of how the men understood or felt about their military service. Most black soldiers were illiterate, and even if some did acquire a form of literacy while members of the WIRs, writing equipment was expensive and not always in ready supply in remote locations. Thus, we are left with sources written by white people that need to be read with caution and awareness of pre-existing racial attitudes. It is partly for this immensely practical reason that this book focuses on how others perceived and interpreted the men of the WIRs.

As this book will demonstrate, those thinking about race as a concept in the early nineteenth century, how 'blackness' could be defined, measured or quantified as something tangible and in opposition to 'whiteness', turned again and again to the example of the WIRs. As Chapter 1 explains, the entire rationale for the creation of the regiments in the dying years of the eighteenth century rested upon ideas about black bodies and their resistance to tropical diseases that were exacting a heavy toll on white Europeans. During the early decades of nineteenth century, the surgeons attached to the WIRs helped to forge a notion, explored in Chapters 2 and 3, of the 'superhuman' black man, able to undertake physical challenges that were simply beyond the white man. This largely positive view of those of African descent neatly coincides

---

[22] A. B. Ellis, *The History of the First West India Regiment* (London: Chapman and Hall Ltd, 1885); Caulfeild, *One Hundred Years' History*.

with Britain's era of humanitarianism identified by James Walvin.[23] The deterioration in racial perceptions of WIR soldiers occurs almost immediately after full emancipation in the British West Indies was achieved in 1838. Working with a vast array of medical data that compared white and non-white soldiers, military statisticians, discussed in Chapter 4, began to chip away at the idea of the medical supremacy of black soldiers and highlight their vulnerabilities instead. The popularity and pervasiveness of these publications spread far beyond British military or medical circles and had a significant international impact, which is the subject of Chapter 5. By the second half of the nineteenth century, old tropes about black resistance to tropical diseases had almost entirely been replaced by new ones, discussed in Chapter 6, that emphasised the new-found medical vulnerability of black troops, even in tropical zones. Studying the WIRs therefore allows historians to measure the evolution of racial thought in the nineteenth century relating to one specific body of men, where slavery is not the defining issue. Overwhelmingly, the data and discussion of the soldiers of the WIRs deals with them as black men, and not as enslaved black men, even though a number technically were enslaved until 1807. Some writers deliberately went out of their way to draw a distinction between the WIRs and the enslaved or, later, the newly emancipated West Indian population.[24]

Military Medicine

This book is also a medical history, specifically of military medicine in the nineteenth century. It is a history both of surgeons serving with the British army, either attached directly to the WIRs or to the general staff at command headquarters, as well as of medical thought. Hundreds of medically trained personnel served with, or alongside, the WIRs, observing the men up close and first-hand. Some were fresh-faced young men straight from medical school (most frequently graduating

---

[23] Britain's humanitarian spasm occurred between 1787 and 1838, ending with the abolition of slavery in its West Indian colonies. Afterwards, Britain underwent a bout of collective amnesia, claiming the moral high ground for abolition while forgetting about Britain's central role in establishing and driving the slave trade in the first place. James Walvin, *England, Slaves and Freedom, 1776–1838* (London: Macmillan, 1986), 19–20.

[24] For a discussion of the ambiguous legal status of some WIR soldiers, see Roger Buckley, *Slaves in Red Coats: the British West India Regiments, 1795–1815* (New Haven: Yale University Press, 1979), 63–81. The purchased men were all formally emancipated in 1807, though the army had never treated them like slaves – none were sold for example.

from Edinburgh University), others were veterans with many years of prior service with white regiments. Civilian doctors already based in the West Indies were sometimes drafted in to assist the army, particularly during wartime. One historian of military medicine has described an appointment to a WIR as the 'shortest straw' any up-and-coming physician could draw, but that characterisation is a little unfair.[25] In the eighteenth and early nineteenth centuries, the West Indies was the most likely place where army physicians would gain experience overseas during active operations.[26] And some of these physicians turned out to be the most eminent medical minds of their day, publishing widely and holding high office in the Army Medical Department. Surgeons serving with the WIRs dealt with every ailment that the men presented with, from the minor to the life-threatening, and arguably, since on average every man visited the hospital at least once a year, surgeons knew more of the men than any other single white officer.

Surgeons kept detailed records of every case they treated, noting symptoms, possible diagnoses, attempted treatments and eventual outcomes. These records were reported back to London, both in tabular form (where they would be used to collate vast quantities of medical statistics) and with an accompanying narrative. Since they spent a great deal of time trying to treat illnesses that, with hindsight, we know they had no means of curing, surgeons read treatises and medical journals that offered advice on the latest treatments. Occasionally they would contribute their own articles, highlighting regimens they considered particularly effective. Sometimes they published books on diseases common among armies or the possible cures for tropical fevers. Their experiences were inevitably shaped by their day-to-day encounters with mainly African-born men, but what made their writings particularly interesting to those beyond the army was that they often contrasted

---

[25] Marcus Ackroyd, Laurence Brockliss, Michael Moss, Kate Retford and John Stevenson, *Advancing with the Army: Medicine, the Professions, and Social Mobility in the British Isles, 1790–1850* (Oxford: Oxford University Press, 2006), 157, 165.

[26] See J. D. Alsop, 'Warfare and the creation of British imperial medicine, 1600–1800', in G. Hudson (ed.), *British Military and Naval Medicine, 1600–1830* (Amsterdam: Rodopi, 2007), 23–50; R. L. Blanco, 'The development of British military medicine, 1793–1814', *Military Affairs* 38 (1974), 4–10; Michael Joseph, 'Military officers, tropical medicine, and racial thought in the formation of the West India Regiments, 1793–1802', *Journal of the History of Medicine* 72 (2017), 142–65; Suman Seth, *Difference and Disease: Medicine, Race and the Eighteenth-Century British Empire* (Cambridge: Cambridge University Press, 2018), 94; Katherine Paugh, 'Yaws, syphilis, sexuality, and the circulation of medical knowledge in the British Caribbean and the Atlantic world', *Bulletin of the History of Medicine* 88 (2014), 227; Mark Harrison, *Medicine in an Age of Commerce and Empire: Britain and Its Tropical Colonies, 1660–1830* (Oxford: Oxford University Press, 2010), 3–14.

their treatments for black soldiers with those for white officers or, if working in a garrison hospital, with ordinary white rank and file soldiers. There were very few medical environments in the early nineteenth century where black and white bodies were treated side by side, allowing surgeons to observe the ways in which the two responded differently to treatment. The cumulative weight of this unique literature began to shape wider debates about black and white bodies, and later influenced discussions about the different 'races' of humanity.[27]

This book builds on the work of several scholars who have highlighted the link between the publications of army surgeons and the shaping of racial ideas in the eighteenth and early nineteenth centuries. Mark Harrison, for example, observed that physicians based in the West Indies, many of whom had associations with the military, 'had an important bearing upon the development of ideas about race and susceptibility to disease'.[28] John Rankin's study of the British in West Africa in the nineteenth century acknowledged that 'race was an important part of British military plans in West Africa', determining the composition of garrisons for instance, while Suman Seth's exploration of medicine and race in the British Empire in the eighteenth century makes repeated use of the publications of military physicians to demonstrate how they helped to shape early racial attitudes.[29] These works, despite being excellent contributions to the wider field, make little, or in some cases no, use of the extensive records relating to the WIRs. Indeed, several fail to acknowledge that some of the most important military-medical writers of the eighteenth century, including Benjamin Moseley and Robert Jackson, served alongside black soldiers at some point during their careers. Rana Hogarth's engaging and informative *Medicalizing Blackness* does deal briefly with the WIRs, but then moves swiftly on to a broader discussion about diseases believed to be peculiar to enslaved people in the United States.[30] In short, this book aims to

---

[27] For an excellent discussion of this relating to the eighteenth century, see Erica Charters, 'Making bodies modern: race, medicine and the colonial soldier in the mid-eighteenth century', *Patterns of Prejudice* 46 (2012), 214–31. See also Catherine Kelly, *War and the Militarization of British Army Medicine, 1793–1830* (London: Pickering and Chatto, 2011), 11; and Wendy D. Churchill, 'Efficient, efficacious and humane responses to non-European bodies in British military medicine, 1780–1815', *The Journal of Imperial and Commonwealth History* 40 (2012), 137–58. Churchill's otherwise excellent article is let down by a failure to make use of War Office and Colonial Office papers in the UK National Archives.

[28] Harrison, *Medicine in an Age of Commerce and Empire*, 108.

[29] John Rankin, *Healing the African Body: British Medicine in West Africa, 1800–1860* (Columbia: University of Missouri Press, 2015), 135; Seth, *Difference and Disease*.

[30] Rana A. Hogarth, *Medicalizing Blackness: Making Racial Difference in the Atlantic World, 1780–1840* (Chapel Hill: University of North Carolina Press, 2017).

delve much deeper into the rich sources relating to the WIRs and place them at the heart of the evolution of racial ideas from the late eighteenth century onwards.

The West Indies

The Caribbean acts as a backdrop to this study. For more than a century, between 1492 and the early seventeenth century, the Spanish dominated the Greater Antilles, undertaking what can perhaps best be termed a genocide against the native Taino peoples.[31] From the 1620s first the English and then the French, Dutch and Danes successfully challenged the Spanish monopoly in the Caribbean, establishing their own colonies and commencing nearly two centuries of tit-for-tat island conquests that eventually saw Britain emerge with the most profitable island possessions in 1815. The Caribbean was crucial to the formation of British racial ideas because it brought light-skinned British people into close, regular and sustained contact with dark-skinned African people for the first time. Although the British explored a large part of the world in the seventeenth century, incorporating much of it into the British Empire, the West Indies was the only tropical region to see significant immigration from the British Isles. The direction of British settler migration in the 1600s was definitely westwards, first towards Ireland, then across the Atlantic to the Americas. Commercial enterprise in Asia, by contrast, often revolved around trade with powerful and populous states, with permanent British settlement often limited to coastal factories.[32] In Africa only a very small number of British people attempted to reside in the slave-trading forts in Sierra Leone or at Cape Coast castle.[33] The most profitable opportunities in the Americas lay not in trading with native peoples, but in the production, processing and exporting of staple crops, tobacco in the Chesapeake and sugar in the West Indies. This necessarily involved the settlement of people willing and able to clear land and plant crops. The most important of the early British Caribbean colonies was Barbados, first settled in 1627, which rapidly attracted a resident landowning planter class, and a far

---

[31] Tink Tinker and Mark Freeland, 'Thief, slave trader, murderer: Christopher Columbus and Caribbean population decline', *Wicazo Sa Review* 23 (2008), 25–50; Gad Heuman, *The Caribbean: a Brief History*, 2nd ed. (London: Bloomsbury, 2014), 7–16.

[32] Emily Erikson, *Between Monopoly and Free Trade: the English East India Company, 1600–1757* (Princeton: Princeton University Press, 2014), 51–76.

[33] Philip D. Curtin, *The Image of Africa: British Ideas and Action* (Madison: University of Wisconsin Press, 1964), 9.

larger mass of white indentured servants to work on the land. Indeed, for all the dominance of New England and the Chesapeake in the historiography of early America, twice as many British people migrated to the West Indies than the North American mainland in the first half of the seventeenth century.[34]

It was not long, however, before white indentured servants began to be supplanted by African slaves. By the time Jamaica was wrested from Spanish control in 1655, there was little attempt to experiment with white labour and the focus was on importing as many Africans as possible for sugar cultivation. The shift from white indentured labour to black enslaved labour was not immediate, but once the transition began it was unstoppable.[35] A number of interlacing factors influencing the growth of slavery were at play simultaneously in the West Indies, but most historians agree that economic considerations were paramount. The supply of indentured servants began to dry up at the same time that the number of Africans imported by English ships, long involved in the transatlantic slave trade, was rising. For English planters, who co-opted the entire legal basis of slavery from the Iberian powers, the economic equation became straightforward: over the *longue durée* it was far cheaper to import Africans, who might provide twenty or more years of labour as well as future generations of workers via natural reproduction, than use white indentured servants on fixed-term contracts.[36]

Largely absent from historiographic discussion about the transition from white indentured to black enslaved labour in the West Indies is any sense that the impact of tropical climates on the human body was relevant. No one attempted to justify or rationalise the enslavement of black people in the seventeenth century by claiming that only those used to a tropical climate could work in such heat. After all, white servants had been employed successfully, though no doubt uncomfortably, in

---

[34] About 80,000 British migrants went to the West Indies before 1650, compared to about 40,000 to the North American mainland. Between 1651 and 1675, numbers of migrants were roughly comparable at 65,000–70,000 each. After 1675, however, West Indian migration tailed off sharply compared to North America. Alison Games, 'Migration', in David Armitage and Michael J. Braddick (eds.), *The British Atlantic World 1500–1800* (New York: Palgrave, 2002), 41.

[35] Hilary Beckles dates the changeover to c. 1690, but a little earlier in Barbados. Hilary McD. Beckles, 'A "riotous and unruly lot": Irish indentured servants and freemen in the English West Indies, 1644–1713', *William and Mary Quarterly* 47 (1990), 505.

[36] For the historiography on the origins of slavery and the interplay of racial and economic factors, see among others, Jordan, *White over Black*; David Eltis, *The Rise of African Slavery in the Americas* (Cambridge: Cambridge University Press, 2000); Betty Wood, *The Origins of American Slavery: Freedom and Bondage in the English Colonies* (London: Hill and Wang, 1998), 48–51; Dunn, *Sugar and Slaves*, 73.

Barbados in the first half of the seventeenth century. Yet the Caribbean was absolutely central to the formation of British ideas about tropical climates in general.[37] As James Lind pointed out in the mid-eighteenth century, there was a professional opportunity 'for medical observations, during a very sickly season in the West Indies, when thousands of Europeans are sent thither at once'.[38] The hot climate was obviously alien to the British, it was usually the first thing that new arrivals noticed, and therefore most physicians thought it would inevitably have a negative medical impact.[39] As one Barbadian doctor remarked, heat and moisture combined to 'render the fibres of the body more lax, abate the vigour of the circulation, increase the viscidity of the blood, promote sensible, and diminish insensible perspiration'. These rapid physical changes had consequences that manifested as a 'seasoning' fever, indeed 'there are very few upon their first arrival who escape the attacks of this furious invader ... the fatality of this disease deservedly place[s] it in the front of destroyers'.[40] The experience of John Taylor, who visited Jamaica in 1687, was perhaps typical. Within weeks of his arrival twenty-two-year-old Taylor succumbed to a fever that reduced him to 'perfect weakness' for more than three weeks. After a lengthy convalescence he was then 'violently seized' with a stomach illness.[41] Taylor was a short-term visitor to the West Indies, but permanent immigrants surviving the seasoning fevers were not by any means guaranteed a healthy future since the periodic appearance of new diseases put everyone in danger. In 1692 a 'terrible contagion ... raged like a pestilence' in Barbados, killing up to twenty people per day in Bridgetown, with the high mortality attributed to the fact that the disease 'probably derived from the coast of Africa'.[42] The disease was most likely yellow fever, and a further outbreak in Kingston, Jamaica, in 1737 killed a quarter of the

---

[37] As David Arnold and Mark Harrison have pointed out, ideas about the climate of the West Indies helped to shape how the British viewed the climate of the Indian subcontinent. David Arnold, 'India's place in the tropical world, 1770–1930', *The Journal of Imperial and Commonwealth History* 26 (1998), 1–21; Harrison, *Climates and Constitutions*.

[38] James Lind, *An Essay on Diseases Incidental to Europeans in Hot Climates* (London: T. Beckett, 1768), 121. See also Seth, *Difference and Disease*, 104–9.

[39] Arnold, 'India's place in the tropical world, 1770–1930', 5; David Arnold, 'Race, place and bodily difference in early nineteenth-century India', *Historical Research* 77 (2004), 254–73; Charters, 'Making bodies modern', 227.

[40] Richard Towne, *A Treatise of the Diseases Most Frequent in the West Indies* (London: John Clarke, 1726), 11, 19.

[41] David Buisseret, *Jamaica in 1687: the Taylor Manuscript at the National Library Jamaica* (Kingston: University of the West Indies Press, 2000), 29–31, 39.

[42] Edmund Burke, *An Account of the European Settlements in America* (London: R. J. Dodsley, 1760), II, 88.

population.[43] Perhaps most frightening of all, there was little anyone could do to avoid illness. Even those taking every precaution were 'by no means secure'.[44] The hostile disease environment took a heavy toll on migrants to the West Indies. Trevor Burnard has demonstrated that deaths far outnumbered births in Jamaican parish registers and that even in the eighteenth century more than a third of indentured servants died within five years of arrival.[45]

The 'seasoning' fevers combined with other exotic and particularly deadly epidemics to create, to use Karen Kupperman's phrase, a 'fear of hot climates' in British minds.[46] This fear was exacerbated by what David Arnold has termed a 'great outpouring' of medical publications that outlined in often graphic detail just how pestilential such illnesses could be for Europeans.[47] These publications should have terrified anyone contemplating a voyage to, let alone permanent settlement in, the West Indies. Keen followers of writings about the Caribbean would have been unable to avoid the overwhelming impression that 'the climate of the West Indies [is] unfriendly and unpleasant to an European constitution'.[48] No doubt most migrants to the Caribbean expected to become sick on arrival, but they came anyway spurred on by the enormous potential for riches beyond imagination. Servants completing their term of indenture hoped to obtain lands of their own, something few would have aspired to in England or, if not, a comparatively high-waged position. The demand for skilled white workers remained persistently high throughout the seventeenth and eighteenth centuries.[49] And there was always the dream that, with a huge helping of good fortune, the seasoning process would work. Mark Harrison and Suman Seth have pointed out that eighteenth-century medical writers generally agreed that European settlers could, eventually, adapt sufficiently to live safely in the tropics. Most believed that as humans

[43] Trevor Burnard, 'Not a place for whites? Demographic failure and settlement in comparative perspective, 1655–1780', in Kathleen E. A. Monteith and Glen Richards (eds.), *Jamaica in Slavery and Freedom: History, Heritage and Culture* (Barbados: University of the West Indies Press, 2002), 81.

[44] Hugh Smythson, *The Compleat Family Physician or, Universal Medical Repository* (London: Harrison and Co., 1785), 479.

[45] Burnard, 'Not a place for whites?', 80.

[46] Karen Ordahl Kupperman, 'Fear of hot climates in the Anglo-American colonial experience', *William and Mary Quarterly* 41 (1984), 213–40.

[47] Arnold, 'India's place in the tropical world, 1770–1930', 5.

[48] Burke, *An Account of the European Settlements in America*, II, 96. Harrison, writing mainly about India, dates this fear to the nineteenth century, but it is clear that it also existed in the eighteenth century largely based on information from the West Indies. Harrison, *Climates and Constitutions*, 9–10.

[49] Burnard, 'Not a place for whites?', 75–6.

shared a common origin, and had spread across the globe to populate torrid, temperate and frigid zones, it was self-evident that adaption was possible. There were plenty of white individuals who had survived for twenty or thirty years in Barbados, St Kitts, Antigua and Jamaica who were living proof.[50] Becoming acclimated was a lottery, however, and mortality of new migrants remained stubbornly high.

If white mortality was appalling then, if anything, enslaved mortality was worse. Although the theory of climate held that the natural inhabitants of a hot climate were not white, they were black, imported Africans singularly failed to thrive in the West Indies.[51] A number of explanations can be proffered – Africans were often sick when they arrived; planters cut costs by reducing provisions, clothing and shelter for enslaved people (compared to white indentured servants), leading to increased vulnerability to disease due to malnutrition or exposure; and it was simply cheaper to replace overworked slaves with new arrivals than spend resources maintaining those already there.[52] For those who bothered to comment, and many did not, high mortality among enslaved people was usually attributed to 'excessive labour', not to the climate and not to the tropical fevers that so decimated white immigrants.[53]

Embodied Differences

Although it was widely accepted that climate was responsible for physical differences among men, and that fair-skinned men lived in cold regions while dark-skinned men lived in warm regions, West Indian physicians in the eighteenth century actually thought these differences to be quite superficial. Since 'human bodies are greatly influenced by the climate, air, soil, diet etc of the places we inhabit', it was inevitable that the skin tones of enslaved Africans and their European enslavers would be different, but, according to Barbadian Richard Towne, 'this reaches no deeper than the outward cutis'.[54] Most believed there was little or no underlying physical dissimilarity between whites and blacks. Griffiths Hughes, whose *Natural History of Barbados* was published in 1750, reported that

---

[50] Harrison, *Climates and Constitutions*, 9, 11, 91; idem, *Medicine in an Age of Commerce and Empire*, 64; Seth, *Difference and Disease*, 3, 93–4.

[51] On the tenacity of this belief, despite it being clear that Native Americans and Africans residing at the same latitudes did not have the same skin tone, see Jordan, *White over Black*, 14.

[52] Carl and Roberta Bridenbaugh, *No Peace beyond the Line: the English in the Caribbean 1624–1690* (New York: Oxford University Press, 1972), 354–5; Dunn, *Sugar and Slaves*, 313–14; Betty Wood, *The Origins of American Slavery*, 50–1.

[53] Burke, *An Account of the European Settlements in America*, II, 124.

[54] Towne, *A Treatise of the Diseases*, 1. See also Seth, *Difference and Disease*, 74, 192.

he 'never could find out any extraordinary difference' between white and black bodies, and that even their mental abilities were broadly similar, taking into account education.[55] And while eighteenth-century Caribbean physicians observed varieties in the diseases that white and black people were prone to, they did not generally attribute this to innate differences between white and black bodies, instead pointing to either adaptation or circumstances. Richard Towne's *Treatise of the Diseases Most Frequent in the West Indies*, published in 1726, noted some diseases were more common among black people, but they could also be found in 'white people, whose unhappy circumstances have reduced them to Hardships but little inferior to what the blacks are obliged to undergo'.[56] William Hillary observed that many Barbadian epidemics 'generally seize the negroes first' but mused, 'Is it not because they are little or thin clothed, and often poorly fed, and much more exposed to all the variations of the air, and inclemencies of the weather?' High rates of tetany he attributed to 'the negroes going barefoot, and thereby being more exposed to such injuries ... [or doing] such work as renders them more liable to get such wounds'. Diseases often thought to originate in Africa, such as elephantiasis and yaws, he noted had spread into the white population 'who are not exempted from it'.[57]

Yellow fever was the single exception to the general understanding that diseases were largely indiscriminate. In the seventeenth and early eighteenth centuries, this virulent and deadly disease was confined to tropical regions, though it would eventually venture as far north as New York, Philadelphia and Gibraltar. West Indian physicians quickly noticed that the disease 'most commonly seizes strangers, especially those who come from a colder, or more temperate climate'.[58] Several also observed that 'native white men of the islands are seldom affected' or, at the very least, they seemed to be 'much less obnoxious to it'. But the immunity of local whites was not absolute. Hugh Smythson believed that natives leaving the tropics for any period became vulnerable on their return, and white men engaging in 'debauches or violent exercise' risked becoming ill regardless of their nativity.[59] Whites of all types

---

[55] Griffith Hughes, *Natural History of Barbados* (London: author, 1750), 14, 16.

[56] Towne, *A Treatise of the Diseases*, 188.

[57] William Hillary, *Observations on the Changing Nature of the Air and the Concomitant Epidemical Diseases in the Island of Barbadoes*, 2nd ed. (London: L. Hawes, 1766), 206–7, 227, 305, 339. See also Seth, *Difference and Disease*, 62, 68–9, 78–9, 84–6.

[58] Hillary, *Observations on the Changing Nature of the Air*, 146.

[59] Smythson, *The Compleat Family Physician*, 479. Edward Long was one who claimed that 'the natives, black and whites, are not subject, like Europeans, to bilious, putrid, and malignant fevers'. Edward Long, *The History of Jamaica* (London: T. Lowndes, 1774), II, 534.

certainly seemed to be less immune than Africans, 'none of whom, of either sex, natives or foreigners, are ever known to be attacked by it'.[60] Henry Warren in Barbados was among many medically trained people who struggled to explain how 'the negroes, whose food is mostly rancid fish or flesh, nay often the flesh of dogs, cats, asses, horses, rats etc who mostly lead very intemperate lives, and who are always worse clad, and most exposed to surfeits, heats, colds, and all the injuries of the air, are so little subject to this danger?'[61] Scottish physician Alexander Wilson speculated that 'the continued vegetable diet' of field slaves 'acts as a constant corrector of putrescent tendency', thus exempting them from the disease.[62] The perceived vulnerability of Europeans, and comparative immunity of Africans, to yellow fever would come to lie at the very heart of discussions at the end of the eighteenth century about physical differences between white and black bodies. Was it a case of something innate in the black body that offered greater resistance to this disease, or simply a matter of black bodies being better adapted to the environment? This debate, as we shall see in the following chapter, had a direct influence on the creation of the WIRs.

The West Indies held a peculiar sway in English minds of the eighteenth century. As home to the largest emigrant English population in a tropical region, the Caribbean islands clearly helped to shape and disseminate ideas about how heat affected health. After the loss of the mainland American colonies, it was also the only region that could give emigrant Britons a first-hand encounter with imported African slaves. But, as we have seen, despite a brutal plantation regime that held little regard for the welfare of enslaved people, older ideas about race that emphasised religion, language, technology and civilisation above all were remarkably persistent and had yet to undergo any radical transformation. Black bodies, deep down, were understood to be pretty much the same as white ones. The superiority of white Christian culture was unquestioned, of course, but not because of some innate difference in white biology. Lack of opportunities and education were most often blamed for the supposed inferiority of Africans, rather than inherent flaws with brains or bodies.

In the final decade of the eighteenth century, the Caribbean continued to draw European attention. The uprising of enslaved people in

---

[60] Smythson, *The Compleat Family Physician*, 479.

[61] Henry Warren, *A Treatise Concerning the Malignant Fever in Barbados* (London: Fletcher Gyles, 1740), 13.

[62] Wilson also believed that 'negro domestics, who live much on animal food, are as subject to putrid epidemics as the white inhabitants'. Alexander Wilson, *Some Observations Relative to the Influence of Climate on Vegetables and Animal Bodies* (London: T. Cadell, 1780), 172.

French St Domingue in 1791 had repercussions throughout the Atlantic World, and soon afterwards Britain, France and Spain resumed their long imperial rivalry in the region. Simultaneously, debates in Britain over the morality of the international slave trade to the West Indies highlighted to a wider audience the truly terrible conditions endured by captives. This led some people to begin to question how Europeans treated non-white people more generally. But most importantly for our purposes, it was during this tumultuous decade that Britain would embark on a military experiment, the WIRs, that would eventually help to entirely refashion white ideas about black bodies.

1 Medical Necessity and the Founding of the West India Regiments

On 17 April 1795 Henry Dundas, secretary at war, wrote to General Sir John Vaughan, commander in chief in the Leeward Islands, authorising him 'to raise two corps of mulattoes or Negroes to consist of 1,000 rank and file each'.[1] These were the first of what would become, within just three years, twelve West India Regiments (WIRs) stationed throughout the British Caribbean. The decision to recruit large numbers of black soldiers into the British army seems, at first glance, to be counterintuitive since the entire British Caribbean had been constructed and predicated upon the enslavement and brutal oppression of black bodies. Most persons of African descent living in the West Indies would have experienced physical abuse including, but not limited to, beatings, rape and torture. To even contemplate taking some of these people, giving them weapons and training, required confidence that they would direct their aggression solely against foreign enemies and not on their erstwhile enslavers. Yet despite significant and persistent resistance from white planters, rapidly spreading and increasingly urgent ideas about race, climate and disease resistance combined to create an environment whereby the recruitment of black men into the British army became absolutely essential by 1795.

Military campaigns in the West Indies throughout the eighteenth century had faced an enemy far more deadly than rival European powers. As J. R. McNeil has ably demonstrated, mosquito-borne diseases exerted a significant influence over the imperial history of Caribbean. The best laid plans of generals in London repeatedly fell apart as carefully gathered forces melted away before their eyes.[2] According to John Bell, the surgeon attached to the 94th regiment, 'In every war, during the course of this century, in which the forces of Great Britain have been

---

Dundas to Vaughan, 17 April 1795, WO1/83, UK National Archives. N.B.: All WO (War Office) and CO (Colonial Office) references pertain to volumes in the UK National Archives.

[2] J. R. McNeill, *Mosquito Empires: Ecology and War in the Greater Caribbean, 1620–1914* (Cambridge: Cambridge University Press, 2010), 149–87.

9

employed in the West Indies, it has unfortunately happened, that the number of those who have perished by disease has, in every instance, greatly exceeded the loss occasioned by the sword of the enemy'.[3] John Hunter, who managed the military hospitals in Jamaica between 1781 and 1783, agreed, calculating that 'in less than four years [1777–81], there died in the island of Jamaica 3,500 men; those that were discharged amounted to one half of that number, which make in all 5,250 men, lost to the service in that short period of time, from the climate and other causes of mortality, without a man dying by the hands of the enemy'.[4] The obvious conclusion for these military surgeons was that 'the climate is certainly unfavourable to a British constitution, as it contains the causes of so many diseases, so far peculiar to itself, that those diseases are either not known, or very rarely met with in Britain'.[5] Many considered the most dangerous time to be when a regiment had newly arrived in the West Indies and endured the well-known, but no less dreaded, 'seasoning' fevers. Hunter reported, 'Those who are just arrived from cool and healthy climates, are particularly subject to fevers, as is daily experienced by all new comers. A regiment always loses a greater proportion of men the first year than afterwards'.[6] The seasoning process, Edmund Burke remarked, ensured that a new regiment 'can never meet the enemy in the field with much more than half their complement'.[7] Serving with the army in the West Indies gained such a notoriety that by 1788 one author claimed it was well-known back in Britain 'that the soldiers sent to the colonies, provided with every necessary, and experiencing the most humane treatment, decrease most rapidly'. As a result, 'out of one thousand men landed in any one of the islands, five hundred shall be dead or non-effectives in twelve months'. These were not singular occurrences, it was 'the fate of almost every regiment sent to the West Indies', despite 'every possible care and indulgence'. The unavoidable conclusion was that 'the lives of Europeans are considerably abridged by a long residence under the torrid zone'.[8] Unsurprisingly, some considered it a waste of military

---

[3] John Bell, *An Inquiry into the Causes Which Produce and the Means of Preventing Diseases among British Officers, Soldiers and Others in the West Indies* (London: J. Murray, 1791), 1; see also *London Medical Journal* 3 (1782), 249.

[4] John Hunter, *Observations on the Diseases of the Army in Jamaica* (London: G. Nicol, 1788), 70–1.

[5] Bell, *An Inquiry into the Causes*, 8.

[6] Hunter, *Observations on the Diseases*, 23.

[7] Edmund Burke, *An Account of the European Settlements in America* (London: R. J. Dodsley, 1760), II, 119.

[8] Joseph Woods, *Thoughts on the Slavery of the Negroes* (London: for the author, 1788), 11–12.

resources to transport and maintain large white garrisons in the West Indies 'who die and waste away without any benefit to themselves or their country'.[9] Few in Britain looked upon military service in the West Indies positively.

Reading the observations of military surgeons from the 1780s, it would be easy to assume that mortality rates for British regiments approached 50 per cent. However, using the muster rolls of regiments stationed in the West Indies, David Geggus calculated that between 1764 and 1786 death rates among British soldiers arriving in the West Indies averaged 14.5 per cent in the first year and 6.6 per cent in subsequent years. Of course, an additional number were sick, and perhaps had to be invalided from service, but this still did not approach anything like 50 per cent.[10] By the mid- to late 1790s, regimental surgeons would actually look back on the 1780s as a remarkably healthy period. With their opinion undoubtedly coloured by the terrible loss of life that occurred after 1793, the level of mortality during the 1780s was now accepted as tolerable. John Weir, in charge of the military hospital in Jamaica, stated that in the 1780s 'the troops were in general healthy, and although fevers were frequent, they were not fatal'. Theodore Gordon in Barbados in the early 1790s agreed: 'The troops I served with enjoyed a high degree of health, especially those corps in which a good system of interior economy was established and preserved; the mortality was very small'.[11] Even John Hunter admitted that there were posts in Jamaica, especially 'elevated and mountainous situations', where 'the proportion of deaths was altogether inconsiderable'.[12] This led William Pym, looking back in 1848, to claim, rather unrealistically, that troops based in the West Indies before 1793 enjoyed 'as high a degree of health as in any part of Europe'.[13]

While the actual military impact of high rates of sickness and mortality among regiments in the West Indies prior to 1793 was debatable, it was never sufficient to seriously threaten British control of its possessions for example, it was clear that much of the blame could be attached to the climate and particularly the various tropical fevers that did not exist in Britain. Numerous medical authorities in the eighteenth century had firmly established the negative impact that a tropical

[9] Burke, *An Account of the European Settlements*, II, 120.
[10] David Geggus, *Slavery, War and Revolution: the British Occupation of Saint Domingue, 1793–1798* (New York: Oxford University Press, 1982), 364.
[11] Sir William Pym, *Observations on Bulam, Vomito-Negro or Yellow Fever* (London: John Churchill, 1848), 51–2.
[12] Hunter, *Observations on the Diseases*, 32–3.
[13] Pym, *Observations on Bulam*, 55.

climate would have on the health of a newly arrived person from a temperate zone. Military surgeons read the same medical texts as their civilian counterparts and quickly agreed that fevers impacted the various populations in the West Indies differently, with those of African descent tending to prove highly resistant. John Hunter in Jamaica was not alone in thinking that 'the negroes afford a striking example, of the power acquired by habit of resisting the causes of fevers; for, though they are not entirely exempted from them, they suffer infinitely less than Europeans'. Hunter was, of course, referring to the belief that those of African descent were able to become perfectly acclimated to a tropical climate, so much so that even those who resided 'in the marshy parts of the country [were] very little subject to the fever'. Whites, 'after remaining some time in the West Indies', he thought, also became 'less liable to be affected by the causes of fevers'.[14] Although Hunter does not provide hard evidence to support his conclusions, there is a subtle difference in his descriptions of comparative immunity. Whites could become 'less liable' via the seasoning process, whereas blacks 'suffer infinitely less'. This suggests that even among seasoned populations, he believed fever affected whites more than blacks. Yet despite the fact that white vulnerability and comparative black immunity to tropical fevers was a popular theory long before the 1790s, voices advocating a permanent alteration in the composition of British military forces in the region were extremely scarce.

Black soldiers in the British army were not a sudden novelty in 1795. The creation of the WIRs was actually the culmination of several decades of evolving British military policy in the Caribbean. Roger Buckley, whose 1979 monograph *Slaves in Red Coats* remains the best study of the early years of the WIRs, highlights the demographic equation that made military reliance on whites in the Caribbean impossible. West Indian islands had very small white populations, barely sufficient to form a small militia if required for defence, and certainly not large enough to repel a determined assault from an invader. The preferred solution for much of the eighteenth century was the periodic co-option of enslaved men to bolster island militias. This was a perfectly logical choice and could be seen as an extension of the system of slavery that dominated the West Indies.[15] The elite white men who sat in the island assemblies were accustomed to controlling the bodies of black people, using them however they saw fit, and therefore had every reason to use

[14] Hunter, *Observations on the Diseases*, 24, 192.
[15] Roger Norman Buckley, *Slaves in Red Coats: the British West India Regiments, 1795–1815* (New Haven: Yale University Press, 1979), 2–6.

enslaved men to make up for a deficiency in military manpower. The militia units were under local control, indeed white planters themselves served as militia officers and would thus be supervising their own slaves. Surrendering enslaved men to the authority and control of an outside body, such as the British army, was an entirely different matter but it actually occurred on several occasions during the eighteenth century.

Most white West Indians would have agreed with Edward Long 'that the Negroes, so far from suffering any inconveniences, are found to labour with most alacrity and ease to themselves in the very hottest part of the day'.[16] It is therefore not too surprising that the army had, in a piecemeal fashion, been recruiting enslaved men in small numbers since at least the 1740s, using them as 'pioneers' to undertake arduous physical labour for the army. More than 400 participated in the Cartagena expedition of 1740, ostensibly to 'perform such Drudgery as the Heat of the Climate made difficult for Europeans', but it was not long before commanders on the ground 'thought proper to arm most of these people, and to employ them in Night parties to reconnoitre, and disturb any Parties the Enemy might have sent out with the same Intention'.[17] During the siege of Havana in 1762, the army eventually obtained via purchase or hire about two thousand enslaved men for military use. Since regimental surgeons recommended 'all drudgery and labour should be performed by negroes, and others, inured to the climate', the weaponry and ammunition for the siege was hauled into place by '500 blacks purchased ... at Martineco and Antigua for that purpose'.[18] Once the city had been captured, army commanders were no doubt grateful of the black auxiliaries as within weeks half of the white troops fell sick. In each instance, black men were not formally embodied into regiments but instead simply attached to white regiments in small groups, and, significantly, they were dispensed with once the campaign was over. Hired slaves were returned to owners, purchased slaves were sold.

[16] Edward Long, *History of Jamaica* (London: T. Lowndes, 1774), II, 412.
[17] Maria Alessandra Bollettino, '"Of equal or of more service": black soldiers and the British empire in the mid-eighteenth-century Caribbean', *Slavery and Abolition* 38 (2017), 514; see also McNeill, *Mosquito Empires*, 149–68.
[18] Bollettino, 'Of equal or of more service', 521; Erica Charters, 'Making bodies modern: race, medicine and the colonial soldier in the mid-eighteenth century', *Patterns of Prejudice* 46 (2012), 229; Elena A. Schneider, *The Occupation of Havana: War, Trade, and Slavery in the Atlantic World* (Chapel Hill: University of North Carolina Press, 2018), 126–8; Benjamin Moseley, *A Treatise on Tropical Diseases on Military Operations,* 2nd ed. (London: T. Cadell, 1789), 184; Patrick Mackellar, *A Correct Journal of the Landing His Majesty's Forces on the Island of Cuba; and of the Siege and Surrender of the Havannah, August 13, 1762* (London: Green and Russell, 1762), 6; Stephen Conway, 'The mobilization of manpower for Britain's mid-eighteenth century wars', *Historical Research* 77 (2004), 385.

The most that the commander of the Havana expedition would do for 'the Negroes that were bought for the Crown at Antigua' was to order them 'to be sent to some of the British Colonies to be dispos'd of as it would be a hardship to sell them to the Spaniards contrary to their own Inclinations'.[19] There was no suggestion that the men who had served the army would be freed. Although auxiliary military roles, such as portering, kitchen duty, ditch-digging and latrine duty, became the norm for these men, some in the West Indies began to see a possible future need for a permanent establishment of black soldiers. Edward Long recommended in 1774 that in order to prevent 'the French or Spaniards from making conquest of our island', up to 10,000 'of the more sensible, able, and trusty' slaves should be armed and intermixed with the white regiments and used 'particularly in nocturnal surprizes, harassing skirmishes and ambuscading'.[20] Long's idea did not go any further, but it was clearly not forgotten.

The event that helped more than anything else to crystallise ideas about how differently white and black soldiers reacted to tropical illnesses was the expedition of 1,800 white regular troops, together with black auxiliaries, that the British army mounted against Fort San Juan in Nicaragua in 1780. Thomas Dancer, physician to the forces, confirmed that all 'those sent upon service … were at the time of our departure in general good health'.[21] Soon after besieging the fort, however, a large number of the number of white soldiers fell sick, and matters did not improve once the fort was taken. Hoping to secure good barracks where the sick could be treated, Dancer instead described the fort as 'calculated only for the purpose of breeding infection'.[22] Benjamin Moseley, who also accompanied the expedition, reported: 'none of the Europeans retained their health above sixteen days, and not more than 380 ever returned, and those, chiefly, in a miserable condition. It was otherwise with the Negroes who were employed on this occasion; a very few of them were ill, and the remainder of them returned to Jamaica in as good health as they went from it'. The same difference in susceptibility to disease was apparent during the short-lived occupation of Fort Omoa in Honduras: 'On that expedition, half the Europeans who landed, died in six weeks. But very few negroes; and not one, of

[19] Instructions to the Honourable William Keppel, 25 December 1762, CO117/1.
[20] Long, *History of Jamaica*, 133, 135; James Lind, *An Essay on Diseases Incidental to Europeans in Hot Climates*, 4th ed. (London: J. Murray, 1788), 143.
[21] Thomas Dancer, *A Brief History of the Late Expedition against Fort San Juan, so far as It Relates to the Diseases of the Troops* (Kingston: D. Douglass and W. Aikman, 1781), 8.
[22] Ibid., 19.

200, that were African born'.[23] Moseley is arguing here that simple possession of black skin provided protection against tropical fevers, with only a slightly diminished level of immunity afforded to those of West Indian rather than African birth. The significant contrast he draws is between anyone with black skin and 'Europeans', by which he meant any white person, not just those newly arrived from Europe. The expedition included 200 creole volunteers from Jamaica as well as detachments from the 60th and 79th regiments. Dancer made a similar point regarding Amerindian allies, observing that 'Cape Indians, who had an admixture of negro blood' proved less prone to sickness than other local people.[24]

The first conclusion that many drew from the Nicaraguan expedition was that 'sickness will prevent European troops succeeding... where the service exceeds six weeks'.[25] The second was that the British should look seriously at using black troops more systematically. John Hunter's residence in Jamaica came more than a decade after Edward Long's, but it is quite likely he read the *History of Jamaica* since he closely followed Long in recommending that throughout the Caribbean 'there should be a certain number of negroes attached to each regiment; or what perhaps would be better, a company of negroes and mulattoes should be formed in every regiment, to do whatever duty or hard work was to be done in the heat of the day, from which they do not suffer, though it would be fatal to Europeans'.[26] Significantly, it is clear that ideas about the climatological suitability of those of African descent to West Indian service began to circulate in London through the published writings of military surgeons such as Moseley and Dancer.[27] British ministers would thus have had an awareness of the inhospitable Caribbean climate, and particularly its impact on the strength of white regiments stationed there, several years before the WIRs were founded in 1795.

The idea of using black troops periodically resurfaced in the decade following the failed Nicaraguan expedition. Alex Dirom, adjutant general to the governor of Jamaica, believed an easy way to augment

---

[23] Moseley, *A Treatise on Tropical Diseases*, 134.
[24] Ibid., 78; and Dancer, *A Brief History*, 12.
[25] Moseley, *A Treatise on Tropical Diseases*, 181.
[26] Hunter, *Observations on the Diseases*, 36.
[27] Michael Joseph rightly stresses the importance of ground commanders in the decision to form the West India Regiments who, after all, reported the ever-decreasing strength of their forces on a monthly basis, but he overlooks the writings of medical personnel in the years before 1795. Michael Joseph, 'Military officers, tropical medicine, and racial thought in the formation of the West India Regiments, 1793–1802', *Journal of the History of Medicine* 72 (2017), 142–65.

the island's military forces with 'the strongest and most active people' would be for slave owners to bring a few 'trusty' slaves with them to the regular musters 'to be trained and disciplined in the militia'.[28] In 1787 Lieutenant John Gosling, then serving with the 1st Regiment of Foot in the Caribbean, even outlined a scheme to the foreign secretary for recruiting a corps of 'free mulattoes and blacks' precisely because they were 'inured to the climate, [and] are not subject to those diseases so fatal to Europeans'. These men would be 'ever ready for any service' and in particular for 'all duty of fatigue which must ever be, as was the case in the last war in the West Indies, fatally destructive to our soldiery until they become reconciled to the climate'.[29] Unlike Moseley, Gosling retained a hope that white soldiers might become seasoned in time, but there was clearly a growing chorus of voices suggesting that black troops would be a positive addition to British military forces in the West Indies.

One fully fledged unit of black soldiers was actually stationed in the British Caribbean before 1795. Although small, and usually overlooked by historians, the Carolina Corps demonstrated just how effective black troops could be in the West Indies. The Carolina Corps, as the name suggests, had been created in the latter stages of the American Revolutionary War in South Carolina. Fugitives from slave plantations 'attached themselves' to the army and were eventually given weapons and even mounted in order to strike terror among patriots. As the war drew to a close in 1782, British commanders faced calls to return these fugitive slaves as part of the evacuation agreement. But, aware that 'many of them, which had taken an active part, had made themselves so obnoxious to their former owners' and now faced 'the severest punishment', army commanders instead decided to relocate 300 of them to St Lucia and, importantly, to retain them as a military unit. In 1783 they were posted to garrison Grenada, newly restored to Britain by the Treaty of Paris, where they were 'to assist in doing the laborious duties' of rebuilding fortifications and military buildings. Additionally, they were deployed against fugitive slaves on the island and 'found more useful, than the other troops, from being better able to bear fatigue in that climate'.[30]

---

[28] Alex Dirom, *Thoughts on the State of the Militia of Jamaica Nov. 1783* (Jamaica: D. Douglass and W. Aikman, 1783), 14.

[29] John Gosling to the Marquis of Carmarthen, c. October 1787, British Library Add MS 28062 (f.378) in the correspondence of the 5th Duke of Leeds v.3, 1787. See also F. Guerra, 'The influence of disease on race, logistics and colonization in the Antilles', *Journal of Tropical Medicine and Hygiene* 49 (1966), 34.

[30] 'Of the Carolina, or Black Corps, serving in the Leeward Islands', CO101/31. See also Gary Sellick, 'Black skin, red coats: the Carolina corps and nationalism in the revolutionary British Caribbean', *Slavery and Abolition* 39 (2018), 459–78.

General Edward Mathew, commanding in Grenada, pushed strongly in late 1790 and early 1791 for the Carolina Corps to be doubled in strength and to be given a central role in the military structure of the Leeward Islands command. He readily dismissed fears about the loyalty of armed black men in a slave society as having 'no weight; as experience shews they are not only to be depended upon, but are more inveterate against people of their own colour, than any other troops'. But he based the main thrust of his argument on the greater medical value of black soldiers compared to whites. He estimated 'loss of soldiers in the West Indies, by death, or rendered useless to the service by the climate' at 10 per cent per annum, three times that of the Carolina Corps. Moreover, each black soldier was 'known to be capable of doing more work for a continuance, than Europeans in that climate'.[31] Recruiting more black soldiers, either volunteers from among black loyalists settled in Nova Scotia or via purchase, who could undertake 'the duties most unfriendly to European constitutions... would probably save the lives of many soldiers, and certainly add much to the comfort, convenience and durability of the troops'.[32] Nativity was evidently not thought to be that important; black men born in mainland North America, the West Indies or Africa were all equally suitable. The home secretary in London, Lord Grenville, thought Mathew's plans were 'very desirable' and instructed that 'no opportunity should be lost of enlisting Negroes, or people of colour, to keep that corps as complete as possible'.[33] An attempt was subsequently made to recruit in Nova Scotia, not least because 'a great number... had been employed as Pioneers' during the Revolutionary War' and thus were already accustomed to military life. However, only sixteen new recruits resulted from this mission, despite existing Carolina Corps soldiers being dispatched to explain the benefits of enlistment. Mathew attributed his failure to the simultaneous arrival of an alternative, and ultimately far more attractive, offer from the Sierra Leone company that did not require the men to leave their families and friends behind.[34]

At the same time that he was learning of the important role of the Carolina Corps in the Leeward Islands from General Mathew, Grenville was requesting the governor of Jamaica, the Earl of Effingham, to consider 'the means of raising black troops in the colony, either as separate

---

[31] 'Of the Carolina, or Black Corps', CO101/31.
[32] Matthew to Grenville, 22 December 1790, CO101/31.
[33] Grenville to Matthew, 8 March 1791, CO101/31.
[34] Mathew to Grenville, 1 March 1791, CO101/31; Mathew to Dundas, 14 January 1792, CO101/32.

corps, or to be attached as additional companies to the regiments'. At a time when war with Spain looked increasingly likely, Grenville considered this to be a 'point of considerable importance, particularly with a view to offensive operations'.[35] By October 1790 Grenville told Effingham he had consulted with General Adam Williamson, commander of forces on the island, and they had agreed that 'it seems particularly desirable that a number of Negroes or people of colour should immediately be embodied. ... The utility of a body of men of this description, particularly with a view to the preserving the health of the European troops, when on service, is likely to be very great, that I cannot too strongly recommend it'.[36] Grenville was effectively acting as the conduit between the Leeward Islands command and the Jamaican command. Evidence and ideas from General Mathew in Grenada, who had an active black corps under his command, were being filtered via London to General Williamson in Jamaica. Grenville recommended that in the first instance free blacks should be recruited, with planters 'contributing' their slaves 'as an aid to Government' if insufficient free blacks were enlisted. If both of these sources failed to provide enough men to form one company per regiment stationed in Jamaica, then Grenville recommended 'purchasing on the public account a number of Negroes for this object'. Anticipating the objections that would be raised from Jamaican planters 'on many accounts', Grenville nevertheless believed that 'the advantages appear to be so very great, both as a substantial augmentation of effective force, and of affording the means of preserving the lives of the British soldiers, that I am extremely anxious to see it, if possible, carried into effect without delay'.[37]

The stage had clearly been set for the formation of more units of black soldiers in the West Indies, but when the threat of war with Spain receded in 1790 these plans lost their urgency. Grenville still thought the idea 'would probably be of great advantage to the service if executed to a limited extent', and General Williamson agreed. There were only two choices available to those holding a Caribbean command he thought: either leave European troops on their ships 'as the only sure means of avoiding the diseases of the climate', or embody 'a very considerable corps of blacks'. The latter course was 'absolutely necessary' if any offensive operations were planned.[38] By early 1791 Williamson acknowledged that the peace between Britain and Spain 'renders the measure at present unnecessary', but Grenville confided to Effingham that he was

[35] Grenville to Effingham, 10 July 1790, CO137/88.
[36] Grenville to Effingham, 6 October 1790, CO137/88.
[37] Ibid.
[38] Williamson to Grenville, 14 November 1790, CO137/89.

'inclined to believe that even under the present circumstances of peace, it will be highly advisable to adopt some plan ... in order to preserve the health of the European troops'.[39] Effingham agreed that the establishment of a corps of 400 men who could be used in small detachments where needed would be extremely useful.[40] What is apparent in these conversations is a clear shift from a military to a medical rationale for black troops. The military threat from Spain might have dissipated, but the inhospitable climate remained unchanged.

The plan for recruiting black soldiers was still being discussed when the first reports of the slave uprising in St Domingue arrived in Jamaica in September 1791. The destruction wrought just over a hundred miles away by armed black men, 'who have burnt and destroyed all the plantations for 50 miles in length on both sides [of] the cape', quickly ended any attempt to raise a black corps in Jamaica.[41] Mathew's plan to increase the establishment of the Carolina Corps in Grenada also came to nought, and their numbers continued to decline steadily.[42] Planter complaints that arming black men was both foolish and dangerous suddenly seemed prescient and evidently far outweighed a desire to reduce mortality among European troops. Even annual regimental mortality rates of 10 per cent were acceptable in the effort to avoid facilitating another St Domingue.

Fears about the havoc armed black troops might wreak, of course, did not diminish the reality of an unfavourable disease environment in the West Indies for white soldiers. Throughout the early 1790s military commanders continued to lament that high mortality rates among white regiments made their jobs more difficult. Lieutenant Colonel Sir William Myers, commanding at Prince Rupert's Head in Dominica, reported in September 1791 that 'both artillery and the 60th regiment are exceedingly unhealthy; their hospital full, and the men dying daily, their disorder a fever of the intermittent kind'. Prince Rupert's Head was one of the best defensive sites in the entire West Indies. Jutting

---

[39] Williamson to Grenville, 19 December 1790; Grenville to Effingham, 7 January 1791, CO137/89.

[40] Grenville to Effingham, 7 January 1791; Effingham to Grenville, 19 March 1791, CO137/89.

[41] Effingham to Dundas, 7 September 1791, CO137/89. Some have sought to depict the creation of the WIRs as a response to the revolt in St Domingue, whereas the opposite was clearly true: it stopped initial plans in their tracks. G. M. Orr, 'The origin of the West India regiment', *Journal of the Royal United Service Institution* 72 (1927), 129–30.

[42] George F. Tyson, 'The Carolina black corps: legacy of revolution (1782–1798)', *Revista/Review Interamericana* 5 (1975/6), 661–3. By 1794 Vaughan claimed only 'about a hundred' of the Carolina Corps were fit for duty, though there were 213 men actually listed as members. Vaughan to Dundas, 25 December 1794, WO1/83. Monthly return January 1795, WO17/2486.

into the ocean and dominated by two large hills with commanding views of the sea route between Martinique and Guadeloupe, the Board of Ordnance declared Prince Rupert's 'the only one in the Leeward Islands worthy of consideration as a place of arms'. The problem was that the landward side, abutting the fort at Prince Rupert's, was mainly swamp and a perfect breeding ground for mosquitoes that spread tropical diseases. But while the fort experienced high rates of both mortality and debilitating sickness, to the extent that Myers could 'scarcely find men to do the ordinary duties of the post', he stopped short of recommending the use of black soldiers instead. Even General Mathew, who forwarded Myers's letters to London, and who had enthusiastically championed black soldiers just a year before, was now silent on the issue. St Domingue had changed everything, and radical solutions were off the table. High rates of sickness were simply to be expected and endured in the West Indies, unhealthy posts could be found throughout the islands and became something to work around. In this instance Myers suggested stationing troops elsewhere in Dominica and only bringing them to Prince Rupert's during periods of military alarm.[43]

What forced British commanders in the Caribbean, and their political masters in London, to reconsider the use of black soldiers was the outbreak of a particularly virulent strain of yellow fever in 1793. The virus was transported from Bolama Island off the coast of Guinea-Bissau in West Africa in July 1792 by the ship *Hankey*.[44] The *Hankey* had led an idealistic British colonisation effort in Africa that sought to demonstrate that slavery did not have to be the defining paradigm of European encounters with Africans. Instead, these colonists wished to establish a colony based on free labour, with native Africans being paid for any work they did. Their idealism proved to be misplaced, partly because of the mistrust of locals who had experienced several centuries of European incursions. What rapidly destroyed the colony, however, was disease. Within weeks of arriving on Bolama Island, the first colonists began to fall ill. On 19 July only six out of eighty-six colonists were reported as sick; thereafter the proportion of sick grew as the numbers of colonists steadily declined. At the end of August, fifteen of the sixty-six remaining colonists were sick; at the end of October, thirty-four of fifty-three survivors were sick – many of whom evidently did not recover. By the end of November, all but one of the twenty-seven

---

[43] Myers to Mathew, 4 and 19 September 1791, in Mathew to Dundas, 10 October 1791; see also Mathew to Dundas, 2 November 1791, CO101/31.

[44] For a thorough account of the *Hankey*'s voyage, see Billy G. Smith, *Ship of Death: a Voyage That Changed the Atlantic World* (New Haven: Yale University Press, 2013); Geggus, *Slavery, War and Revolution*, 352.

remaining colonists were ill with fever, and by the end of January 1793, only thirteen were left alive.[45] Not all colonists died of disease, some fled the island to take their chances on the mainland, but the majority succumbed to yellow fever, an endemic disease in tropical climates that is found throughout West Africa. What made 'Bulam fever' particularly dangerous was that it had evolved on an island uninhabited by humans, with only monkeys as hosts. It proved to be far deadlier than the regular strains of yellow fever.[46]

The Bolama strain of yellow fever would probably have remained in Africa but for the *Hankey*. The ship was anchored off the island between July and November 1792, giving plenty of time for a local colony of *Aedes aegypti* mosquitoes, responsible for spreading yellow fever, to establish themselves on the ship. In November and December 1792, the ship meandered around the West African coast before heading first for the Cape Verde islands and then the West Indies. The *Hankey* arrived in Barbados on 14 February 1793, before swiftly moving on first to St Vincent on 16 February and Grenada on the 19 February, where it would remain until July.[47] Cases of yellow fever did not appear immediately of course. Mosquitoes from the ship first had to bite an uninfected person such as a customs inspector or crewmember from a ship moored alongside, and it took several days for symptoms to appear. And for the epidemic to become established in the town, the local population of urban *Aedes aegypti* had themselves to become vectors by feeding on an infected person, a process that can take up to two weeks.[48] Nevertheless, once introduced the virus spread inexorably and would continue until there were no more susceptible humans. Colin Chisholm, surgeon to His Majesty's Ordnance in Grenada, documented the spread of a 'very fatal fever', first to the ships moored closest to the *Hankey* in harbour of St George's, then to those a little farther away. By mid-April the first cases appeared on shore and thereafter the disease became truly epidemic. Chisholm estimated that about two-thirds of the population of

---

[45] Philip Beaver, *African Memoranda Relative to an Attempt to Establish a British Settlement on the Island of Bulama* (London: C. and R. Baldwin, 1805), 104, 130, 159, 181, 190.

[46] On monkeys as a repository for yellow fever, see Smith, *Ship of Death*, 69, and McNeill, *Mosquito Empires*, 49–50. On yellow fever more generally, see Andrew Spielman and Michael D'Antonio, *Mosquito: a Natural History of Our Most Persistent and Deadly Foe* (New York: Hyperion, 2001), and Christopher Wills, *Yellow Fever – Black Goddess: the Coevolution of People and Plagues* (Reading: Addison-Wesley, 1996).

[47] Beaver, *African Memoranda*, 471.

[48] When temperatures average 25°C, mosquitoes can pass on the virus after fourteen days, but at 30°C they can pass it on after just ten days. Michael A. Johansson, Neysarí Arana-Vizcarrondo, Brad J. Biggerstaff and J. Erin Staples, 'Incubation periods of yellow fever virus', *American Journal of Tropical Medicine* 83 (2010), 183–88.

St George's became infected and that of those about a fifth perished.[49] Regiments stationed in Grenada also succumbed, partly due to their own incautious behaviour. Some members of the 45th regiment, stationed closest to the *Hankey*, visited the somewhat notorious ship out of 'curiosity'. Several soldiers subsequently died, and not only did they take the virus back to their barracks, they also unwittingly transmitted it to visiting friends from other regiments. Worst affected were twenty-seven new recruits for the Royal Artillery who arrived on Grenada in mid-July. By the middle of August, twenty-one of them were dead.[50]

The virus spread quickly throughout the Caribbean islands. The harbour of St George's was full, and some ships probably departed for other ports, taking either infected mosquitoes or humans with them, before the extent of the epidemic became fully known. Others fled in a vain attempt to escape the pestilence. The governor of Grenada ruefully noted that the 'constant communication' between islands meant that the spread of the disease was 'almost unavoidable'.[51] A significant factor in the spread of yellow fever was the slave revolt in St Domingue that had created a tsunami of refugees. Some fled St Domingue for other Caribbean islands where the epidemic had already taken hold, but ships also brought the virus to St Domingue itself, meaning those leaving the island often took infected people to previously uninfected regions. It was those fleeing St Domingue who brought yellow fever to Philadelphia in the fall of 1793.[52] Another critical aid to the spread of the disease was the outbreak of hostilities between Britain and France in early 1793. The movement of troops between the various British islands in preparation for assaults on Guadeloupe and Martinique ensured that no island was spared this deadly virus.

Yellow fever had, of course, been a regular visitor to the Caribbean for more than a century, but it had been just one of a variety of tropical fevers, including malaria, that affected newly arrived Europeans. From 1793, however, this highly virulent strain of yellow fever took centre stage. In the first three months of the outbreak on Dominica,

---

[49] Colin Chisholm, *An Essay on the Malignant Pestilential Fever Introduced into the West Indian Islands from Boullam, on the Coast of Guinea, as It Appeared in 1793 and 1794* (London: C. Dilly, 1795), 82–95. Ninian Home, the governor of Grenada, first mentioned the epidemic in a letter dated 2 May 1793, CO101/33.

[50] Chisholm, *An Essay on the Malignant Pestilential Fever*, 95–6, 98.

[51] Home to Dundas, 16 July 1793, CO101/33.

[52] On Philadelphia, see J. H. Powell, *Bring Out Your Dead: the Great Plague of Yellow Fever in Philadelphia, in 1793* (Philadelphia: University of Pennsylvania Press, 1949), and Billy G. Smith and J. Worth Estes, '*A Melancholy Scene of Devastation*': the Public Response to the 1793 Philadelphia Yellow Fever Epidemic (Philadelphia: Science History Publications, 1997).

for instance, Dr James Clark recalled the impact on newly arrived St Domingue refugees: 'eight hundred emigrants, including their servants and slaves, were cut off by this fever. ... Few newcomers escaped an attack, and very few of those recovered'. No wonder that local physicians believed it to be 'as quick and fatal as the plague'.[53] The high mortality also began to be noticed in Britain. Whitehall officials naturally received communiqués from both island governors and military commanders, but such was the havoc caused by this outbreak that occasional reports also surfaced in the British press. In August 1793 the London *Times* reported that 'the plague, brought from Bulam, which first made its appearance at Grenada, has spread most alarmingly. Eighty persons died in one day at Grenada of this disease'.[54] In early 1794 reports circulated that 'during the last six months Grenada, Tobago, St Vincent's and Dominica have lost, on the most moderate calculation, one third of their white inhabitants, principally by the yellow fever'.[55] Yet the outbreak did not dominate the British press by any means. Indeed, far more accounts were printed of the impact of yellow fever in Philadelphia than in Britain's West Indian islands. This can perhaps be explained by an unwillingness to advertise just how weak British control in the Caribbean actually was when the French were poised to take advantage.

Almost immediately military physicians noted that this strain of yellow fever followed other tropical fevers in affecting white people far more than black people. Observing the disaster unfolding in Grenada, Colin Chisholm commented, 'It is curious, and may be useful, to observe the gradation of this fatal malady, with respect to the various descriptions of people exposed to its infection. Neither age nor sex were exempted from its attack; but some were more obnoxious to it than others, and the colour had evidently much influence in determining its violence'. Chisholm rated the most vulnerable to be sailors and soldiers, especially those 'least accustomed to the climate' or 'lately from Europe'; then white civilians, with those 'lately arrived' most likely to fall sick; followed by mixed-race people, black people and finally children 'especially those of colour'.[56] Interestingly, Chisholm makes no mention of the role that seasoning might have on black people and he

---

[53] James Clark, *A Treatise on the Yellow Fever as It Appeared in the Island of Dominica in the Years 1793–4–5–6* (London: J. Murray, 1797), 2; Chisholm, *An Essay on the Malignant Pestilential Fever*, 102; William Wright, *Memoir of the Late William Wright* (Edinburgh: William Blackwood, 1828), 372.

[54] *Times*, 13 August 1793.

[55] *Bury and Norwich Post*, 1 January 1794.

[56] Chisholm, *An Essay on the Malignant Pestilential Fever*, 99–101.

clearly thought that even seasoned whites were more vulnerable to this disease than any black person. And the darker the skin, the more protection was afforded. Physicians in the West Indies were puzzled by this. William Wright, who served first in Jamaica and then as director of military hospitals in Barbados, recorded that 'people of colour, and negroes, are in a manner totally exempt from this disease' but could proffer no plausible explanation – 'that field negroes should not be liable to it is to me inexplicable'.[57] William Pym, who would become one of the leading experts on yellow fever, was equally bemused as to its selectivity: 'Why it should attack whites in preference to blacks? Why it should prefer a robust European to a languid Creole? And why it should respect the sable race of the West Indies, yet attack the negroes of North America?'[58] These questions would tax the finest medical minds of the age throughout the nineteenth century.

Skin colour was thus pointed to by many as a key factor in determining vulnerability to the disease, yet it was not an absolutely guarantee of immunity, as Wright and some others noted. The medical explanation for the selective impact of yellow fever is largely straightforward. Yellow fever was endemic in West Africa, a zone effectively bounded by the Sahara in the north and the Kalahari Desert in the south, and generally manifested itself as a comparatively mild childhood disease. Native West Africans therefore usually gained lifelong immunity from future infections because of a childhood illness, and obviously retained that immunity if enslaved and transported to the Caribbean. Children born to enslaved parents in the Americas might also have been infected with yellow fever during infancy, since the virus was certainly present if not continuously then at least fairly frequently throughout the eighteenth century, and therefore gained the same immunity as their parents.[59] As Rana Hogarth has pointed out, this acquired immunity was widely interpreted as being innate by medical practitioners because they did not recognise the relatively mild childhood illness as yellow fever.[60] The error is entirely understandable since it bore little resemblance to the violent and often fatal version that affected adults. The small number of

---

[57] William Wright, 'Practical observations on the treatment of acute diseases, particularly those of the West Indies', *Medical Facts and Observations* 7 (1797), 8–9.

[58] William Pym, *Observations on Bulam Fever Which Has of Late Years Prevailed in the West Indies, on the Coast of America, at Gibraltar, Cadiz and Other Parts of Spain* (London: J. Callow, 1815), 154.

[59] Kenneth F. Kiple and Virginia H. Kiple, 'Black yellow fever immunities, innate and acquired, as revealed in the American South', *Social Science History* 1 (1977), 419–36.

[60] Rana A. Hogarth, *Medicalizing Blackness: Making Racial Difference in the Atlantic World, 1780–1840* (Chapel Hill: University of North Carolina, 2017), 41–3.

white children born in the Caribbean were also able to acquire immunity to yellow fever in the same manner.

Yet the thought processes of physicians were muddled by the fact that the virulent strain of yellow fever that arrived in the West Indies in 1793 did not completely exempt black people. In Dominica James Clark noted that while 'the negroes who had been long in the town, or on the island escaped ... the new negroes who had been lately imported from the coast of Africa were all attacked by it. I knew a lot of twenty-four fine healthy new negroes all seized with this fever about the same time, one third of whom died in the course of the disease'.[61] In Martinique 'every person of colour, black as well as mulatto, seemed to suffer from fever', while in Guadeloupe the fever 'was violently contagious, and very few escaped it; even the negroes, who have been considered very unsusceptible of fever, were attacked with it'.[62] The fact that significant numbers of people of West African descent were infected suggests that the Bolama strain of yellow fever was not only new but also different enough from the commonest strains to re-infect people of African origin, even when they had survived a previous bout of yellow fever. Chisholm was adamant that this 'malignant pestilential fever' was not the same as the usual West Indian yellow fever, despite the fact that it shared many of the same symptoms, simply because of higher mortality rates and the rapidity with which the disease killed. In reality the Bolama virus was indeed yellow fever, just a more aggressive and deadly strain. African immune systems, however, effectively had a head start in tackling the new infection and so were far more likely to prove robust enough to defeat it. The consensus view among physicians remained that if black people were not entirely immune, they continued to demonstrate greater resistance to yellow fever than whites, and therefore they possessed an essential biological advantage. This is a key point: immunity was not absolute but comparative, and closely associated with black skin. Chisholm in Grenada recorded that when 'the disease began to appear among the negroes of the estates in the neighbourhood of town ... [it] did not spread much among them, nor was it marked with the fatality which attended it when it appeared among the whites'. He estimated 'that only about one in four was seized with it; and the proportion of its mortality was still more trifling, viz, one to 83'.[63] Europeans, who were far less likely to have acquired immunity, suffered acutely from this more dangerous strain, with mortality rates upwards of 30 per cent.[64]

[61] Clark, *A Treatise on the Yellow Fever*, 2–3.
[62] Pym, *Observations on Bulam Fever*, 13, 118.
[63] Chisholm, *An Essay on the Malignant Pestilential Fever*, 97.
[64] Ibid., 102.

The impact on the British regiments stationed on the various islands was immediate and severe. These soldiers were nearly all born in Europe and few would have had a previous encounter with yellow fever. It is very likely that none had acquired immunity. Surgeon Thomas Reide recalled, 'The army in St Lucia suffered a great deal from sickness; and hardly an officer or private soldier escaped. The mortality was very great'.[65] William Pym, serving with the 70th regiment in Martinique, recorded that 'after the appearance of fever in Grenada in 1793, every station for troops, however healthy before, suffered severely from the contagion'. Using the muster rolls for each regiment, Pym documented the destruction wrought on the army by yellow fever. In 1794 the 9th regiment in St Kitts lost 118 men, the 15th regiment in Dominica lost 93 men, the 13th regiment in Jamaica lost 136 men and the 66th regiment in St Domingue lost 249 men. The 69th regiment lost 313 men within six months of arriving in St Domingue in 1795. These were exceptional losses, far above the usual mortality in the West Indies which just a few years previously had been estimated at about 10 per cent per year. The 9th regiment, for instance, had lost only seventeen men in the six years between 1787 and 1793 and would have been considered a 'seasoned' regiment able to withstand a tropical climate. The fact that this new strain of yellow fever took a heavy toll on regiments that had been in the region for years set alarm bells ringing in London since it challenged the entire premise of 'seasoning'.[66]

With hindsight the decision by the British to invade St Domingue in September 1793 in the midst of a yellow fever epidemic was disastrous. Despite initial gains made in partnership with French royalist planters, the army struggled from the outset with 'that never-failing attendant on military expeditions in the West Indies, the yellow or pestilential fever [which] raged with dreadful virulence'.[67] In what some historians have suggested was a deliberate strategy, black generals such as Toussaint L'Ouverture retreated to the mountains and allowed the yellow fever virus to decimate the enemy.[68] Further outbreaks of yellow fever in 1794, and 1795 in particular, devastated newly arrived regiments. David Geggus has estimated that more than 12,000 British soldiers perished in the five years of the St Domingue campaign. At one point, between August and December 1794, regiments were losing 10 per cent of their men each month. Not all the deaths were caused by

[65] Thomas Dickson Reide, *A View of the Diseases of the Army in Great Britain, America, the West-Indies and On Board of King's Ships and Transports* (London: J. Johnson, 1793), 191.
[66] Pym, *Observations on Bulam Fever*, 128, 130–2.
[67] Bryan Edwards, *An Historical Survey of the French Colony in the Island of St Domingo* (London: John Stockdale, 1797), 149.
[68] McNeill, *Mosquito Empires*, 250.

yellow fever, the regular illnesses that followed armies were no doubt present as well, and malaria was endemic in the region.[69] One French planter glumly informed the Duke of Portland, 'The small detachments of troops which you send out from time to time are not even sufficient to supply the ravages of disease'.[70] The debilitated state of those who had survived yellow fever left regiments incapable of offensive operations. In late summer 1794 General Williamson reported, 'We were, from the great illness and mortality among the troops at St Domingue, obliged to postpone all further operations till after the hurricane months are past, and reinforcements can arrive'.[71]

The rapid spread of the new strain of yellow fever among British troops quartered in St Domingue's ports proved especially devastating. *Aedes aegypti* is an urban mosquito, often travelling just a few hundred metres during its entire life cycle, thriving where people congregate in a comparatively confined area.[72] It is therefore unsurprising that soldiers stationed in Port-au-Prince 'dropt like the leaves in autumn', and all this 'without a contest with any other enemy than sickness'.[73] One military surgeon stationed in St Domingue observed that 'our hospitals contain our garrisons, and the few who carry on duty are languid and convalescent; they are not fit for enterprize or hazard; and nominal armies will never achieve conquests'.[74] Spurred by the example of the French who had enlisted the support of many thousand former slaves, and with operations 'unfortunately crippled by the unprecedented sickness prevailing among His Majesty's naval and military forces', British commanders in St Domingue began recruiting small numbers of local 'negroes to be embodied and to act against the Brigands'. By 'brigands' they meant, of course, the mass of formerly enslaved people fighting for their freedom.[75] By late 1794, 400 black pioneers had been recruited and were 'performing all the most active and laborious services' for the regiments, which, it was hoped, 'would contribute in no small degree, to preserve the health of the regular troops'.[76]

---

[69] Geggus, *Slavery, War and Revolution*, 359, 362, 365–6; David Geggus, 'The cost of Pitt's Caribbean campaigns, 1793–1798', *The Historical Journal* 26 (1983), 699–706.

[70] Malouet to Portland, c. 20 September 1794, WO1/59.

[71] Williamson to Dundas, 1 August 1794, WO1/60.

[72] McNeill, *Mosquito Empires*, 40–44.

[73] Bryan Edwards, *The History, Civil and Commercial of the British Colonies in the West Indies* (London: John Stockdale, 1801) v.3, 174; Edwards, *An Historical Survey*, 164.

[74] Hector M'Lean, *An Enquiry into the Nature, and Causes of the Great Mortality among the Troops at St Domingo: with Practical Remarks on the Fever of That Island; and Directions, for the Conduct of Europeans on Their First Arrival in Warm Climates* (London: T. Cadell, 1797), 40.

[75] Dundas to Williamson, 10 February 1795; Dundas to Williamson, 7 October 1794, WO1/60.

[76] Dundas to Williamson, 6 November 1794, CO1/60.

The consensus of medical professionals in St Domingue was that the only possible path to victory against those native to the island was 'by an army of negroes, possessed of the same habits as themselves, but more expert in arms, and led on by such a proportion of European troops as might animate and encourage them'. Hector M'Lean, assistant inspector of hospitals in St Domingue, believed that had this strategy been adopted early in the campaign it 'would have produced the most beneficial effects; the lives of thousands, who have fallen, not by the sword of the enemy, but by the climate, would have been spared; and the conquest of the island would become more certain and more rapid'. M'Lean was convinced that the embodiment of black soldiers as regular troops would 'more effectually...diminish the mortality of British soldiers in St Domingo...than all the medical exertions of the most experienced and skillful physicians'.[77]

The situation was terrible in St Domingue and has attracted scholarly interest because of its concentration in one place, but the army fared no better elsewhere in the Caribbean. Indeed, more British soldiers perished in Dominica, Grenada, St Lucia and other Windward and Leeward Islands than in St Domingue. General Charles Grey was forced to postpone one planned attack on a French island, garrisoned by 'four thousand blacks and mulattoes in arms', due to the 'sickness and mortality' that prevailed among his own troops. There was, he concluded, 'not even a prospect of success'.[78] Grey repatriated some army units to Britain in late 1794 that were 'very weak, and almost reduced to skeletons', and Grey's replacement in the West Indies, General John Vaughan, found that 'the great sickness and mortality which has prevailed since May last, has broken the strength of all the regiments'.[79] After more than a year of yellow fever whittling away at the army, Vaughan knew that the army would have to scale back its ambitions as 'the whole force in all the islands does not exceed fifteen hundred men', with new arrivals tending to 'fall victim to the climate or are in the hospital before another arrives; this renders me incapable of acting decisively and with vigour'.[80] Vaughan fretted that he did not know 'where this army may look for further reinforcements' since 'the climate will reduce it in some months, to a similar situation in which it now is'.[81]

The desperate situation of the army revitalised the idea of using black troops, and not just in support or auxiliary roles. With his army

[77] M'Lean, *An Enquiry into the Nature, and Causes of the Great Mortality*, 2, 3, 5.
[78] Grey to Williamson, 10 May 1794 in Henry Dundas, *Facts Relative to the Conduct of the War in the West Indies* (London: J. Owen, 1796), 132.
[79] Grey to Portland, 5 November 1794, WO1/83; Vaughan to Portland, 24 November 1794, WO1/31.
[80] Vaughan to Portland, 19 November 1794, WO1/83.
[81] Vaughan to Portland, 24 November 1794, WO1/31.

disintegrating around him, Vaughan came rapidly to 'the opinion that a corps of one thousand men, composed of blacks and mulattoes, and commanded by British Officers would render more essential service in the country, than treble the number of Europeans who are unaccustomed to the climate'.[82] Because of the campaigns against Cartagena, Havana and Nicaragua, those of African descent were already known in military circles to be more resistant to tropical diseases than Europeans, and particularly to yellow fever. Vaughan would have been personally aware of the high mortality among white soldiers during the Nicaraguan campaign of 1780 since it had taken place during his previous stint as commander in the Windward and Leeward Islands. And military surgeons continued to promote the idea of black immunity to the very illness that was dissolving his army. Dr Robert Jackson, who had extensive experience in the West Indies and later became surgeon general of the army, informed the readers of his widely read 1791 *Treatise on the Fevers of Jamaica* that 'it has never been observed that a negro, immediately from the coast of Africa, has been attacked with this disease'.[83] While that claim was modified somewhat by other authors in 1793 as the Bolama strain of yellow fever took hold, the essence of Jackson's point, that black people were far less vulnerable to the disease, remained.

In December 1794, having lost Guadeloupe to a French force consisting of 'four to five hundred whites, and four or five thousand blacks, who are all armed with muskets and bayonets', General Vaughan formally proposed to authorities in London that the army should 'avail ourselves of the service of the negroes' and, significantly, as regular troops 'to be in all respects upon the same footing as the marching regiments'. In purely military terms this made perfect sense: 'as the enemy have adopted this measure to recruit their armies, I think we should pursue a similar plan to meet them on equal terms'. It was simply foolish that 'we have been overlooking the support, which by exertion may be derived from opposing blacks to blacks'.[84] The medical rationale was

---

[82] Vaughan to Portland, 22 December 1794, WO1/31.

[83] The same protection was usually afforded to creole whites, Jackson thought, though he incorrectly believed that anyone, regardless of skin colour, who travelled to 'the higher latitudes of America' or Europe would be susceptible to re-infection on their return to the West Indies. Robert Jackson, *A Treatise on the Fevers of Jamaica, with Some Observations on the Intermitting Fever of America* (London: J. Murray, 1791), 249–50.

[84] Vaughan to Portland, 22 December 1794, WO1/31; Vaughan to Dundas, 25 December 1794, WO1/83. See also Peter M. Voelz, *Slave and Soldier: the Military Impact of Blacks in the Colonial Americas* (New York and London: Garland, 1993), 171, and David Lambert, '"[A] mere cloak for their proud contempt and antipathy towards the African race": imagining Britain's West India regiments in the Caribbean, 1795–1838', *The Journal of Imperial and Commonwealth History* 46 (2018), 630.

actually even more compelling. Black recruits, seemingly unaffected by the epidemics that took such a heavy toll on British regiments, had given the French 'an advantage of the utmost value in this climate', transforming a force of a few hundred into one of several thousand.[85] Vaughan urged the Duke of Portland, who as home secretary had responsibility for the colonies, to take 'into consideration, what great mortality ensues among our troops from the fatigues of service in this climate'. Each British soldier represented an investment of time, training and resources, thus each life preserved was 'saving an extraordinary expence to the nation'. In just a few short months, Vaughan had become 'convinced that unless we can establish and procure the full effect of such a body of men, to strengthen our own troops, and to save them in a thousand situations, from service, which in this country will always destroy them; that the army of Great Britain is inadequate to supply a sufficient force to defend these colonies'.[86] Moreover, military and medical necessity required the units to be properly officered, organised and capable of functioning independently rather than as auxiliaries to white regiments, since it was quite likely that they would be the only healthy regiment at each post.

While awaiting official approval for his plan, Vaughan tried to ensure that white troops 'should be spared on every possible occasion' and therefore dispatched the remnants of the Carolina Corps, now only about a hundred strong, to tackle 'the revolted Negroes at St Lucia ... to endeavour to drive them from their retreat on a mountain', which was deemed 'a proper enterprize on which to employ the blacks, and to save our own soldiers'.[87] He also authorised Captain Robert Malcolm of the 34th regiment to 'raise a considerable number ... [of] mulattoes and blacks, to be on the same footing as the troops of the line ... paying them as troops are paid'.[88] The arguments in favour of black troops were strengthened by a letter written to Vaughan by eight army physicians that he duly forwarded to London. These men 'having had too great occasion to observe the destructive effects of this climate on the health of the soldiers' deplored that 'too many of the soldiers in spite of our best endeavours fall sacrifices to acute disease'. Even those who did not die immediately were left to 'pine away under lingering

---

[85] Vaughan to Dundas, 25 February 1795, WO1/83.
[86] Vaughan to Portland, 24 November 1794, WO1/31; Vaughan to Dundas, 25 December 1794, WO1/83.
[87] Vaughan to Portland, 26 January 1795, WO1/31; Vaughan to Dundas, 31 January 1795, WO1/83.
[88] Vaughan to Dundas, 11 January 1795, WO1/83. Within a month Malcolm had gathered a force of 150 men. January 1795 Return, WO17/2486.

chronic' illnesses because the unhealthy climate was an 'insuperable bar' to recovery. There was no 'seasoning' for British soldiers after 1793, whereby surviving the inevitable bout of sickness during the first few months in the West Indies granted immunity from future illnesses, the disease environment was simply too toxic. Men disembarked, got sick within days, and either died within weeks or remained weak and unable to function as soldiers. The only solution for the sick, they argued, was 'a timely return to a cold climate'.[89] These physicians held out no prospect that white troops would ever thrive in the West Indies.

The weight of opinion from both physicians and military commanders in the West Indies was that medical necessity required a formal and permanent shift in British strategy. It was not that Britain lacked sufficient troops. Time and again in the 1790s, Britain managed to find, equip and train enough men to fight in pursuit of its imperial agenda. There were always jails that could be emptied, or men desperate enough to accept the king's shilling and enlist. Men were not the problem, but finding the right kind of men, particularly for tropical service, proved far harder. When every voice from the West Indies stated clearly that simply sending more troops from Britain was a waste of both men and money, the decision for the government should have been obvious. The voices that gave the government pause came from 'some West India planters and merchants in London'. It is not known exactly what form these representations took, but the West India interest in London certainly acted quickly. Vaughan's letter arrived on Henry Dundas's desk on February 11, and eight days later Dundas replied, telling him to 'refrain from proceeding further in levying Bodies of Negroes to be employed under British Officers, until further signification of his Majesty's pleasure'.[90]

Vaughan received Dundas's 19 February letter on 18 April, and while it was not a definitive refusal to his plan, it was a bitter blow. In his reply, written the same day, Vaughan lamented that 'the enemy avail themselves of the aid, not only of the native white men, but of the negroes who are inured to the climate, can brave the dangers of it, and can so easily be procured in such great numbers, whilst we are confined to the use of European troops, few in number, raw in discipline, and exposed to the

---

[89] Army surgeons to Vaughan, 23 March 1795, WO1/83.
[90] Dundas to Vaughan, 17 April 1795, WO1/83. Dundas references his letter of 19 February 1795 in this April letter but a copy does not seem to be extant. Just a month later Dundas reported receiving 'very pressing representations...from the West India planters' suggesting there was an active line of communication between the West India interest and the government. Henry Dundas to Duke of York, 12 March 1795, WO6/131.

ravages of an unhealthy climate, with which they are unable to contend, and to which they fall such numerous victims'.[91] The imminent loss of the Caribbean colonies would be the result. Indeed, he noted, it was only through the actions of black troops that he had been able to maintain British control of St Lucia and Martinique. Without black troops, however, 'we must remain upon the defensive, which as in this climate, the European troops are constantly diminishing in effectives, will probably lead to more disagreeable consequences'. Vaughan urged the dispatch of more seasoned veterans from Europe because 'it is only filling the hospitals and deceiving yourselves to send out raw, or new raised levies'.[92] One resident of Martinique was dumbfounded: 'How could the merchants of London be so wrong headed as to urge the Duke of Portland to stop General Vaughan from raising and embodying negroes? Never was a step so fraught with mischief to their own interests. We can only be saved by that system. Negroes are employed on all occasions against us, and it is the only strength the enemy have. Believe me, one regiment of negro soldiers is worth, for real service, any two of the British now in the West Indies'.[93] In May Vaughan reported on 'the weakness of our present force which is composed literally of boys and sick men', and confessed 'deep anxiety' about 'the gloomy prospect before me'.[94] The monthly return of military forces in the Windward and Leeward Islands for May 1795 enumerates the scale of Vaughan's problem. From a supposed force of 5,996, only 3,562 were fit for duty, and between 3 and 5 per cent perished each month.[95] Unsurprisingly, with the Caribbean having become 'the inglorious grave of so many thousands', one commentator in London believed 'the military spirit … seems almost extinct'.[96]

Reservations about black regiments among ministers in Whitehall did not last long. Less than two months after ordering a halt to further recruitment efforts, Dundas wrote that after 'a full and deliberate consideration' the government had decided to accept 'the concurrent opinions of almost every officer of rank who has lately been employed in the West Indies', and he told Vaughan to proceed with the plan as quickly as possible.[97] Orders were swiftly out sent from the secretary at war establishing two regiments 'of people of color and negroes' with a 'full complement' of officers 'to be in every respect on the same footing as

---

[91] Vaughan to Dundas Martinique, 18 April 1795, WO1/83.
[92] Vaughan to Dundas Martinique, 28 April 1795, WO1/83.
[93] 'Letter from Martinique May 15', *Gloucester Journal,* 20 July 1795.
[94] Vaughan to Dundas Martinique, 19 May 1795, WO1/83.
[95] May 1795 Return, WO17/2486.
[96] Ronald Hamilton, *Sketch of the Present State of the Army* (London: J. Owen, 1796), 4.
[97] Dundas to Vaughan, 17 April 1795, WO1/83.

the marching reg[imen]ts of inf[antry] on the British estab[lishmen]t'. Each regiment would total more than a thousand men when complete, and a month later orders were issued for six further regiments to be raised.[98] In the intervening period, between initially balking at raising black regiments and granting approval, Dundas had received several letters from Vaughan indicating the effectiveness of informal black militia units that were operating in St Lucia and Guadeloupe.[99] Moreover, the issue was raised in a debate on the slave trade in the House of Commons on 26 February. William Wilberforce pointed out to the administration the weakness of British power in the West Indies ever since the French 'had formed and disciplined them [their former slaves] to the use of arms', and that as a result newly liberated slaves would 'acquire dominion in a climate, where labour, fatigue, and death to our men, were amusement to them'.[100] Alarmist representations from the West India Committee of Planters and Merchants that 'the putting arms into the hands of negro slaves is a measure pregnant with the most fatal consequences' now fell on deaf ears. Even the claim that 'by giving Negroes an establishment as soldiers they would be taught to consider themselves as equal, while they are effectively superior to the whites, as well from their military discipline and skill, as from their numbers' were outweighed by the overwhelming need to provide the army with functional and effective units.[101] Approval from London finally arrived in Martinique on 16 June, providing Vaughan 'much satisfaction'. A letter to Vaughan from General Oliver Nicholls in Grenada, reporting 'the dreadful fever raging here has weakened the militia of the town of St George's so much that I have been obliged to call in two of the militia black compy', completely vindicated his persistence over the recruitment of black troops.[102] Sadly Vaughan's satisfaction was short-lived, he died at the end of July from the same disease, yellow fever, that had rendered his forces so ineffective.

Opposition from colonial legislatures unwilling to provide slaves to the army, as well as the logistical complexity of creating new regiments from scratch, meant that approval from London did not immediately transform the situation. And all the while yellow fever continued to wreak havoc. Major General Paulus Aemilius Irving reported to Henry

[98] Windham to Myers, 24 April 1795; Windham to Fauquier, 27 May 1795, WO4/158.
[99] Vaughan to Dundas, 11 January 1795, 30 January 1795, 31 January 1795 and 25 February 1795, WO1/83. Voelz, *Slave and Soldier*, 133–8.
[100] *Times*, 27 February 1795.
[101] West India Committee Archives, University College London (microfilm), Standing Committee Minutes, 27 June 1795.
[102] Nicholls to Vaughan, 22 June 1795, WO1/83.

Dundas in August 1795 that the army was 'greatly diminished by death, exhausted by fatigue and the disorders incident to this inclement climate', and Vaughan's successor as commander in chief, Major General Charles Leigh, echoed this in October: 'I cannot help lamenting the very distressing state of this army from present sickness and the great loss it has sustained by death'.[103] Even in Martinique, the headquarters of the army in the Leeward Islands and perhaps the most vulnerable to a French counter-attack, one corps had 'nearly three hundred sick out of five hundred and twenty rank and file'.[104] Black recruits into the new WIRs did began to trickle in, mainly from nearby conquered islands. Very few records survive that list the nativity of soldiers from the 1790s, but a list compiled in 1810 of men serving with the 2WIR notes the date they joined. Of twenty-eight black men who had joined in 1795 and survived until 1810, thirteen were from the recently captured French islands of Martinique and Guadeloupe, five were from British islands and a further eight were born in North America. Just two were born in Africa.[105] The only thing these men shared was their black skin, but the problem was that the numbers enlisted were ridiculously insufficient. The 4WIR only had eleven black recruits by the end of 1796, the 6WIR in St Kitts merely nine. Only the 2WIR, with 266 soldiers, was of a useful size.[106]

With the plan to raise black regiments 'having in no way succeeded' and 'not a man having been given by any one of the Islands towards completing them', Leigh co-opted the small informal black militias that had been raised in Dominica and St Vincent by local commanders. At the end of 1796, Soler's Black Corps in Martinique had 318 men, Mears's Black Corps in St Lucia had 487 men and Drualt's Black Corps, also in St Lucia, had 288 men.[107] These men were to be used for 'local and temporary services' since they offered 'considerable advantages... in the present state of the colonies'.[108] Indeed they had already proved their worth by assuming garrison duty in Martinique

---

[103] Irving to Dundas, August 1795, WO1/84; Leigh to Dundas, 2 October 1795. The nadir of effectives occurred in August 1795 with just 2,706 fit for duty. New arrivals from Britain increased the number of effectives but also caused a spike in mortality, in October it reached 6 per cent per month. August and October 1795 Return, WO17/2486.

[104] Leigh to Dundas, Martinique, 8 October 1795, WO1/84.

[105] Even the two Africans might have been in the West Indies some time: one was aged twenty-six and the other twenty-two at the time of enlistment. Succession book of the 2WIR, WO25/644.

[106] 4WIR Succession book, WO25/653; State of the army, December 1796, WO1/86.

[107] Leigh to Dundas, 5 December 1795, WO1/85; State of the army, December 1796, WO1/86.

[108] Dundas to Abercromby, 9 February 1796, WO1/85.

because 'the regiments at Fort Royal and Marin are in a very weak and sickly state'.[109] Faced with 'the failure of the West India Regiments', the army's quartermaster took a decisive step. More than 3,000 black pioneers had been assembled, in line with previous expeditions, to undertake 'common fatigue duties' for Sir Ralph Abercromby's campaign in the Caribbean. The quartermaster decided to arm and equip 758 of them 'to form a body of native troops so essentially necessary in the present war'. This was the largest single arming of black men in the British Caribbean thus far. When added to the existing black troops serving with the Royal Rangers, Guadeloupe Rangers and Dominica Rangers, Abercromby had a force of 1,109 black troops at his disposal. Importantly, when the force gathered in Barbados, only 84 reported sick.[110]

Evidence of the efficacy of the policy of using whatever black soldiers could be found comes from St Lucia. The garrison had been more than 4,000 strong in April 1796, bolstered by the recent arrival of reinforcements under Sir John Moore. The insertion of a large group of non-immunes into an endemic yellow fever zone inevitably led to the disease flaring up again. Shortly after his arrival Moore described the forces under his command as 'perfectly healthy', but within a few weeks, as the transmission and retransmission of the disease via infected mosquitoes began to occur, he noted 'the men begin to fall sick' and the situation thereafter deteriorated rapidly. By the end of August, Moore counted the deaths at 'from sixty to seventy a week'.[111] The commander of Fort Charlotte, overlooking Castries, reported that 'the sickness upon Morne Fortunee and its neighbourhood is dreadful', with 'a bare sufficiency of duty men for the daily guards... so many of the men, are already too ill to be removed; most of those I fear will fall a sacrifice'.[112] Three weeks later the 'dreadful mortality' had spread throughout the forces in St Lucia and Grenada, and 'no abatement whatever has yet taken place in the violence of the disease'.[113] The official record of mortality in the Leeward Islands command between April and October 1796 listed 24,960 hospital admissions in six months, 2,912 of whom perished, mostly in Grenada and St Lucia.[114] Even the medical staff

---

[109] Leigh to Dundas, 5 December 1795, CO1/85.
[110] Return of a brigade of black troops Barbados, 10 March 1796, WO1/85.
[111] J. F. Maurice, *The Diary of Sir John Moore* (London: Edward Arnold, 1904), I, 206, 221, 236.
[112] Moore to [Abercromby?], 19 August 1796, WO1/85.
[113] Graham to Dundas, 9 September 1796, WO1/85.
[114] 'A return of the numbers sick in quarters and in hospitals with those that have died in the Windward and Leeward Charibbee islands since March last', 17 October 1796, WO1/86.

succumbed and commanders were forced to co-opt the services of civilian physicians. By November only just over a thousand men in St Lucia were fit for duty. However, a military census shows a notable difference between white and black troops on the island. Of 344 soldiers from the 31st regiment, for example, just 16 privates were fit for duty, and in total barely a quarter of the white soldiers who remained alive were able to bear arms. By contrast nearly three-quarters of the 775 black soldiers were fit for duty, and they actually formed the majority of fit soldiers on St Lucia.[115] Here was incontrovertible proof that black soldiers had immense value in this toxic disease environment.

Sir Ralph Abercromby, who had assumed command of offensive operations in the Caribbean in 1796, was well aware of 'the many obvious advantages' offered by black troops, particularly when facing 'four thousand black troops at St Lucia' and 'eight thousand well-disciplined troops of colour' in Guadeloupe. As successive regimental returns recorded an ever-diminishing force, with his 12,603 effectives in May 1796 dropping to 8,290 by November and monthly mortality rates nudging 10 per cent, Abercromby's hopes of a rapid and successful military campaign against the French islands dwindled.[116] Reporting to Henry Dundas that 'six British battalions have been nearly annihilated' by what he termed 'the great sickness', Abercromby knew that his only recourse was the 'completion of the Black Corps' as quickly as possible.[117] Continued opposition by local legislatures who refused to provide the men, fearing the 'most dangerous consequences', ultimately forced Abercromby to conclude, 'The Black West India Regts have not gain'd an inch of ground, and there is no prospect of their being completed, unless the negroes are either purchased here, or upon the coast of Africa'.[118] Such a policy would involve expense, 'considerably beyond any calculation hitherto made'; nevertheless, Henry Dundas, accepting the severity of the situation, agreed, authorising Abercromby 'to procure in this manner the number that may be necessary for this purpose'.[119] Dundas was slightly astonished that 'the respective legislatures in so great a proportion of the colonies should have manifested such a decided opposition to a measure supported by the unanimous

[115] Distribution of the forces, 13 November 1796, WO1/86.
[116] May and November Returns 1796, WO17/2487.
[117] Abercromby to Dundas, 16 January 1797, WO1/86.
[118] Abercromby to the Governors of Windward and Leeward Islands, 3 January 1797, WO1/86; Ricketts to Abercromby, 18 January 1797, WO1/86; Abercromby to Dundas, 9 April 1796, WO1/85.
[119] Abercromby to Dundas, 16 January 1797, WO1/86; Dundas to Abercromby, 28 October 1796, WO1/85.

opinion of every officer of rank and experience who has served in the West Indies, proved by the events of this war to be of the most general utility and advantage'.[120] As Roger Buckley has pointed out, the determined opposition of island legislators, in Jamaica especially, stemmed from a desire to preserve existing political, racial and economic structures in the West Indies. The Barbados Assembly, for instance, feared that planters would only give up to the army men 'of the worst characters' and that the French would therefore find it easy 'to turn the arms of these black troops, against the inhabitants of their native spot'. They singularly failed to appreciate the larger imperial view that was taken in London.[121]

Army recruiters tried a number of novel tactics to fill the ranks of the WIRs, including enlisting Irishmen, recruiting in captured French or Dutch islands, poaching the crews of East India Company ships and trawling Chatham docks in England for emigrant West Indians or black Americans.[122] They had some successes. When the 7WIR was disbanded in 1816, more men listed their birthplace as the West Indies than in Africa, the most common locations being Guadeloupe and Curacao, and the 4WIR contained rank-and-file soldiers from Ireland, England, Scotland, Holland, Portugal, India and four different Caribbean islands.[123] Ultimately, however, it was the decision to purchase African men directly from slave ships to augment those already under arms in informal militia units that rapidly increased the number of black troops in the British army. The 4WIR added 244 recruits during 1797 alone, 158 from Africa, with most of the rest from British, French, Danish and Dutch islands, and 3 registering their birth as North America.[124] The one thing that the vast majority of those enlisted shared was black, or at least dark, skin. Non-whites from the West Indies, North America, Africa and even India were all deemed to be similarly suitable, again reinforcing the idea that resistance to tropical diseases was equated with black skin. In September

---

[120] Dundas to Abercromby, 12 May 1797, WO1/86.

[121] Minutes of the Barbados house of assembly, 17 January 1797, enclosed in Ricketts to Abercromby, 18 January 1797, WO1/86. Buckley, *Slaves in Red Coats*, 43–62.

[122] For example, forty-six men born in India were enlisted into the 6WIR in late 1797 and early 1798, all recruited in England. Most (twenty-eight) came from Bengal. This was despite a protest from the directors of the East India Company about the loss of their crews. See Huskisson to Brownrigg, 18 September 1797, WO6/131, and the Succession book for the 6WIR, WO25/657.

[123] WO25/2740 (4WIR) and WO25/2744 (7WIR).

[124] WO25/653 in 1797 listed nativity of new recruits as follows: 158 Africa; 36 St Kitts; 12 Montserrat; 10 St Eustatius; 8 Antigua; 7 Tortola; 3 St Croix; 2 Guadeloupe; 1 Martinique; 1 Jamaica; 1 Nevis; 1 Dominica; 1 St Lucia; 1 New York; 1 Charlestown; 1 America.

1798 Lieutenant General Henry Bowyer had six WIRs in his Windward and Leeward Islands command, totalling 1,551 men. Less than a year later, in July 1799, there were 4,000 men in the WIRs serving in the Windward and Leeward Islands, climbing to 4,640 by 1801.[125]

Agents purchasing slaves for the WIRs were instructed to ensure they were 'of a sound body', with specific height and age criteria, even though the 'age of a negro is not easily known'. All recruits had to be approved as being in good health 'by two of the principal medical staff', who would 'certify the said recruit is unexceptionable'. Higher prices were authorised for a 'seasoned recruit' who had been in the West Indies for a period of time, suggesting that army physicians believed that newly imported Africans would need time to become accustomed to the disease environment, even though they originated from a tropical region and were therefore presumed to already possess a degree of immunity to deadly tropical pathogens. Edward Long had recommended that newly imported slaves should be 'always much indulged during the first two or three years after their arrival, being put to the gentlest work, that they may be gradually seasoned to the change of climate'.[126] Of course, how far planters actually followed this recommendation is debatable, but there was evidently a general belief that despite being highly resistant to tropical fevers, far more so than Europeans, newly arrived Africans would undergo at least a mild form of seasoning.[127] In any event, despite the premium offered for seasoned men, the army found it almost impossible to purchase prime male slaves in the Caribbean. Unseasoned men, straight from Africa, were the only remaining recourse, and by March 1798 General Cornelius Cuyler was 'decidedly of opinion that it is preferable to purchase new negroes, rather than to enlist any who have been for a lengthy time in this country'.[128] But the perils of this shift became obvious within weeks. The governor of Dominica observed that at £56 for each man, 'the contract was too low, and bad negroes were in consequence given'. As a result, 'they are now dying in dozens at Fort George and I am assured of consumption'.[129]

---

[125] Return of the West India Regiments, 6 September 1798, WO1/86; Return of the deaths of the rank and file in the Windward and Leeward Islands, 20 November 1800, WO1/90. Monthly return, March 1801, WO17/2492.

[126] Long, *History of Jamaica*, II, 412.

[127] Realistically, the only viable way to assess whether a recruit was locally born, or had been in the West Indies a while, was by testing their knowledge of a European language. Heads of Instructions, 26 January 1797, Instructions for the officers and medical staff, WO1/86.

[128] Cuyler to Dundas, 8 March 1798, WO1/86.

[129] Cochrane to Dundas, 15 May 1798, Cochrane to Dundas, 7 June 1798, WO1/88.

In reality the problem with those stepping off slave ships was not so much the new diseases they might encounter in the Caribbean, but their poor state of general health on arrival. Being confined below decks on slave ships for several months inevitably resulted in a high mortality rate, approaching 25 per cent in some cases, with dysentery, smallpox and malnutrition taking a particularly heavy toll. Those who, by luck as much as anything else, survived the middle passage certainly did not arrive in the Americas in excellent health. It is therefore hardly surprising that, despite the best effort of army physicians to select only the healthiest individuals as soldiers, it took some time for them to recuperate from the ordeal of the middle passage and that some actually died during the process.[130] There is no way to know for certain how many of the newly purchased slaves never actually donned the uniform of a WIR soldier. Roger Buckley estimated that the Windward and Leeward Islands command purchased 3,992 slaves before the end of 1800. The military returns record 4,559 members of the WIRs by that date, but 1,109 black soldiers had already been embodied by March 1796, before the purchase policy was implemented. The size of the force in March 1796, augmented by purchases, would amount to 5,101, leaving 542 soldiers unaccounted for. The presumption must be that that these men had died before the end of 1800, but no data exists to tell us whether they perished on active service or of disease, nor how many were newly arrived Africans or West Indian creoles.

What became clear very quickly was the massive immunological advantage enjoyed by soldiers of African descent in the West Indies. The earliest data relating to comparative mortality was collected by MP Sir William Young (Table 1.1).[131] The sickness and mortality statistics collated by Young confirmed that the mortality rate for white troops in the West Indies could be as much as tenfold that of black troops and was particularly terrible in 1796, when more than a third of white troops died. Over the ensuing years mortality rates improved for

---

[130] Richard B. Sheridan, 'The Guinea surgeons on the middle passage: the provision of medical services in the British slave trade', *The International Journal of African Historical Studies* 14 (1981), 601–25; Raymond L. Cohn and Richard A. Jensen, 'Mortality in the Atlantic slave trade', *The Journal of Interdisciplinary History* 13 (1982), 317–29; Herbert S. Klein and Stanley L. Engerman, 'Long-term trends in African mortality in the transatlantic slave trade', *Slavery and Abolition* 18 (1997), 36–48.

[131] William Young's father (also Sir William Young) had been the first British governor of Dominica. Young personally visited the West Indies during the 1790s, publishing the *West India Commonplace Book* in 1807. He served as governor of Tobago between 1807 and 1815. R. B. Sheridan, 'Sir William Young (1749–1815): planter and politician, with special reference to slavery in the British West Indies', *Journal of Caribbean History* 33 (1999), 1–26.

Table 1.1. *'Returns of Brit Troops in yᵉ West Indies, from 1795 to 1802 given to W. Y. by J. Sayers Esqʳ Comˢʳʸ [commissary] in yᵉ West Indies',* in Abstract of British West Indian Trade and Navigation from 1773 to 1805

Year	British Troops			Black Corps		
	Force	Dead	Per cent	Force	Dead	Per cent
1796	20,277	7,009	34.6	2,405	75	3.1
1797	14,429	4,145	28.7	2,852	118	4.1
1798	9,989	1,821	18.2	3,058	252	8.2
1799	8,583	1,042	12.1	3,354	258	7.7
1800	9,808	1,387	14.1	4,320	286	6.6
1801	12,785	2,608	20.4	4,604	276	6.0
1802	11,164	1,051	9.4	4,275	299	7.0
Total		**19,063**			**1,564**	

Note: British Library MSS Stowe 921.

whites, mainly due to a dearth of reinforcements from Britain, meaning that white troops who survived a bout of yellow fever had become immune from further infections. Reinforcements in 1800 provided fresh victims for the virus, and mortality rates spiked again at 20 per cent in 1801. In addition to the 19,063 dead, a further 3,065 white soldiers were invalided from the service and sent home to Britain. From a low starting point, mortality rates for black troops rose from 3 to 7 per cent. Young does not provide any information on the causes of increased mortality among black troops. It might readily be accounted for by the rigours of active campaigning, including battlefield injuries, or the appearance of dysentery in makeshift camps, but it remains possible that yellow fever contributed to this rise in mortality as well. It has already been established that while possessing greater resistance to tropical diseases than Europeans, black troops were not completely immune. Such was the virulence of yellow fever in St Domingue that in 1797 'a party of the 5th West Indian regiment, consisting of seventeen men and four officers, the greater part of the men some measure inured to a tropical climate, experienced severe attacks of this fever, (one man excepted), in a residence of less than one month'.[132] But the crux of the issue was the comparative impact on black and white troops. The men of 5WIR might have been sick, but British forces alongside them in St Domingue were so weak they 'could hardly mount a sergeant's guard' and the army completely relied on the 'black corps, [to] occupy

[132] Robert Jackson, *An Outline of the History and Cure of Fever, Endemic and Contagious* (Edinburgh: Mundell and Son, 1798), 71.

all the advanced posts'. Robert Jackson, resident in Port-au-Prince in November 1797 and who observed first-hand the 'blast of pestilence', estimated that about two-thirds of any European garrison would perish from disease each year in St Domingue.[133] The contrast between European regiments and the informal black militias that formed the bulk of the forces under British control in St Domingue was stark: in July 1796 only 224 of 3,491 black soldiers reported sick.[134] Between 1796 and 1802 the average annual mortality rate for black soldiers in the West Indies was 6 per cent, less than a third that of white soldiers at 19 per cent.[135]

Looking back at these statistics in 1807 when he was about to assume the governorship of Tobago, Young tried to suggest that the mortality 'hath yet been exaggerated in the public opinion' and that the West India station had unjustly earned the reputation of a posting of 'almost certain death'. Attributing the extremely high death toll in 1796 to the arrival of troops 'unseasoned to the climate', 'duties of fatigue and service' that were 'immediate and excessive' and 'barracks and hospitals' that were simply 'insufficient' to meet requirements, Young completely failed to mention yellow fever as the principal cause.[136] The disastrous campaign in St Domingue was also conveniently forgotten.

The quantitative and qualitative data available to officials at the time, however, only pointed in one direction – that black troops were far more suitable for West Indian service than whites. A survey of all the WIRs in 1798 listed 83.8 per cent of troops as fit and ready for duty, prompting Henry Dundas to urge commanders in the Caribbean 'to make every possible exertion for the completion of the black regiments and the more particularly so at the present moment as these corps are undoubtedly better calculated for these duties which are so apt to impair the health of European troops when engaged in active service in the West Indies'.[137] General Thomas Trigge, who succeeded Ralph Abercromby as commander in chief in the West Indies, held no hope

---

[133] Williamson to Portland, 6 July 1795, WO1/61; Jackson, *An Outline of the History and Cure of Fever*, 249, 98–9.

[134] General return of foreign and black corps July 1796, WO17/1988. The only WIR soldiers to serve in St Domingue were seconded NCOs serving with the black militia corps. See other returns in WO17/1988.

[135] *Abstract of British West Indian Trade and Navigation from 1773 to 1805*. British Library MSS Stowe 921, p32v.

[136] Sir William Young, *The West-India Common-Place Book* (London: Richard Phillips, 1807), 219.

[137] Return of the West India regiments, 6 September 1798, WO1/86; Dundas to Trigge, 17 May 1799, WO1/87.

that the circumstances for European troops would ever improve: 'The regiments in general have been of late, extremely unhealthy, and many of them so much so, as scarcely to be considered fit for service. The present season has been and still threatens to continue very sickly; our loss already has been considerable, and the prospect before us affords very little hope of amendment'. Trigge was particularly concerned about 'the men who have hitherto escaped illness, are now so much worn down and exhausted from fatigue, as to render it, impossible for them to support it for any length of time'.[138] Dundas once again found himself urging the completion of the WIRs up to their establishment of 500 men each, and using them 'for the preservation of the health of the European troops, by relieving them in those stations which, from the peculiar causes, are found most noxious to their constitutions, and by performing those duties of fatigue to which they are much better adapted than our own troops'.[139] Both statistically by regimental returns, and by the commanders on the ground, the suitability of soldiers of African descent for West Indian service was confirmed.

When John Poyer wrote his *History of Barbados* in 1808, the rationale for the creation of the WIRs was absolutely clear in his mind: 'the extraordinary mortality among the British troops in the West Indies, induced the ministry to adopt the scheme of raising black regiments, who, being inured to the climate, were thought to be better adapted to the service than Europeans'.[140] Increased awareness of black resistance, and white vulnerability, to tropical diseases (particularly yellow fever) was clearly the principal imperative behind the creation of the WIRs. The opposition of local colonial legislatures to armed and trained black men, who might act as an encouragement to the enslaved population to rebel or aid possible French invaders, was overridden by the unanimity of successive commanders in chief in the Caribbean and Home Secretaries in Whitehall. The issue was never insufficient white troops or the distance involved in transporting men from Britain to the West Indies.[141] If those had been the most important factors, then the case would surely have been made much earlier in the eighteenth century for the incorporation of enslaved men into the army. In fact, Britain recruited and shipped tens of thousands of soldiers to the West Indies

---

[138] Trigge to Dundas, 1 August 1800, Trigge to Dundas, 21 August 1800, WO1/89.

[139] Dundas to Trigge, 11 October 1800, WO1/89.

[140] John Poyer, *The History of Barbados from the First Discovery of the Island* (London: J. Mawman, 1808), 624.

[141] On the ability of the army to recruit large numbers at short notice, see Conway, 'The mobilization of manpower', 377–404.

in the 1790s, more than sufficient to achieve their military goals of conquering the French islands. The problem was that the army simply could not keep enough of them alive to do this. The new and virulent strain of yellow fever introduced in 1793 confirmed in military minds the need for a new approach. Amidst much soul searching as to the best way to reduce mortality among white troops, including sending healthier men to begin with, improving diet and accommodation, while reducing rum intake, the solution that ultimately emerged was finding troops who simply did not die in such great numbers. Physicians and surgeons serving in the Caribbean were unanimous that the only men who could do this were Africans.

2   The Ideal Soldier

The WIRs did not immediately emerge as fully formed units in the months following the arrival of approval from London in June 1795. As the previous chapter explained, existing bodies of black troops, often recruited on conquered French islands, were augmented by purchase after 1797 and were amalgamated over several years into actual regiments. At their height, c. 1800–2, there were twelve WIRs stationed all over the Caribbean, with more than 4,500 black soldiers in the Windward and Leeward Islands command alone and further units based in Belize, Jamaica and the Bahamas.[1] For the duration of the war with France, there was little to challenge the medical rationale that had made the embodiment of black soldiers the only logical decision for military commanders and politicians alike. Although mortality in white regiments lessened somewhat during the early years of the nineteenth century, particularly when compared with the devastation of the mid-1790s, medical professionals continued to declare that if white troops were sent to the West Indies, 'in general a great annual sacrifice of even <u>seasoned troops</u> must be the consequence, while unassimilated corps will pay a dreadful tribute to the climate of one half their number in many cases, and always at least one third, before their assimilation is effected'.[2] Looking back in 1817 surgeon William Fergusson neatly encapsulated the standard pattern of Caribbean warfare: British troops successfully captured a French island but 'then the conquest is consecrated by the burial of the troops that achieved it'.[3] Seasoning might lessen the mortality but could not

---

[1] There were 4,640 WIR soldiers listed in the return for the Windward and Leeward Islands in March 1801, WO17/2492.
[2] General return of the sick and wounded…from December 1799 to January 1803, 7–8 CO318/32.
[3] Report to the commander Windward Islands 1817, in William Fergusson, 'On the qualities and employment of black troops in the West Indies', *United Service Journal* (1835), pt 1, 525–6.

eliminate it entirely. One study on troop rotation estimated that if a regiment spent twenty-one of twenty-five years in either the West Indies or India, only 13 per cent of the men originally enlisted would survive to claim a pension.[4] To those at command headquarters, the monthly regimental returns merely confirmed on paper what officers on the ground consistently observed and reported: that white troops continued to suffer far more from disease and illness than black troops. An army report into the outbreak of yellow fever in Philipsburg, St Maarten, in late 1801, where a white regiment suffered 'severely', noted that a detachment of the 4WIR stationed with them 'preserved their usual health during the whole time'.[5] General Thomas Hislop, based in Guyana in 1801, was keen to make his superiors in London aware 'how dreadfully fatal the climate has (in the course of the war) proved to our European regiments ... nor at the present day do we find that the mortality diminishes'. He used the newly arrived 60th regiment in Martinique which 'suffere'd dreadfully' as a salutary example and recalled 'the regiment under my command, was reduced so low at one period (in the year 1798) as to have only a single captain and two subalterns fit for duty'.[6] Data from the early decades following the creation of the WIRs therefore consistently reaffirmed in the minds of those overseeing military affairs, whether in London or the Caribbean, the absolute medical necessity of having black regiments. William Fergusson, well acquainted with the special qualities of black troops having served in St Domingue in the 1790s and in Guadeloupe in 1815, described the WIRs as 'a mine of saving force we had lately opened, and its efficiency and resources can scarcely be over-estimated'.[7] The black soldier was, Fergusson declared, apparently 'fever-proof'.[8] Back in London, James Stephen calculated that 'every black soldier employed in the West Indies saves, in five years, the loss of two European lives at least to the British army'.[9] The military-medical

[4] Alexander M. Tulloch, 'On the relief of corps on foreign service', *United Service Journal* (1836), pt 3, 296.

[5] Nodes Dickinson, *Observations on the Inflammatory Endemic Incidental to Strangers in the West Indies from Temperate Climates Commonly Called the Yellow Fever* (London: E. D. Hewlett, 1819), 181.

[6] 'Hislop's remarks on the establishment of West India regiments written in the year 1801', 4–5 WO1/95. During one the regular inspection of the 6WIR in Dominica, only two white officers were present, 'all the rest at Prince Rupert's having been reported sick'. 6WIR 1812, WO27/113.

[7] William Fergusson, *Notes and Recollections of a Professional Life* (London: Longman, 1846), 206.

[8] William Fergusson, 'On malaria and yellow fever in the West Indies', *United Service Journal* (1837), pt 3, 382.

[9] James Stephen, *Slavery in the British West India Colonies Delineated* (London: Joseph Butterworth, 1824), I, 427.

equation that had driven the forming of the WIRs in 1795 remained basically unchanged and unchallenged through 1815.

The first opportunity to re-assess the purpose and status of the WIRs came when the war in the Caribbean ended in 1815, with some hard-won conquests such as Martinique and Guadeloupe being returned to French control. Unsurprisingly, the number of WIRs shrank as part of a much wider reduction in the size of the army as it transitioned from a wartime to a peacetime establishment. The precedent had been set following the short-lived Peace of Amiens in 1802, when four WIRs had been disbanded.[10] After 1815, a further five WIRs would go and garrison duty would form the principal responsibility of the WIRs in the West Indies from now on. Yet there was never any suggestion that the services of the Britain's black soldiers could be entirely dispensed with. Commanders in the Caribbean and their political masters in London continued to be glad of the resistance that black soldiers offered to tropical illnesses, enabling them to garrison forts in unhealthy places. Some even began to think how they could be used beyond their West Indian base. During the War of 1812 the WIRs had been landed in the United States, in part to deliberately entice the enslaved population to revolt against their owners. In 1814 the 6WIR was present at the burning of Washington, and the 1WIR and the 5WIR fought at the Battle of New Orleans in 1815. Faced with the dilemma of what to do with the fugitive American slaves who had taken refuge with the army following British defeat at New Orleans, Admiral Alexander Cochrane ordered that 'those who choose to adopt a military life, to enlist into any of the WIRs now here'.[11] Cochrane's order is informative. For him, any black man, even those born in the United States, were suitable for the WIRs. Others thought similarly. In 1816 more than 500 black members of the Bourbon Regiment, formed during the British occupation of Reunion Island in the Indian Ocean, were assimilated into the 1WIR.[12] In each case their special qualities were perceived to lie not in nativity, nor in being seasoned to a West Indian climate, but in their darker skin. In the longer term it would not be in the United States, or even in the West Indies, but in Africa that the WIRs ultimately showed their real worth to the British army.

---

[10] The fittest men were transferred from the disbanded regiments to those remaining. For example, the 4WIR absorbed 126 members of the 7WIR, and 39 from the 8WIR in 1802. WO25/653.

[11] Cochrane to Malcolm, 17 February 1815, WO1/143. New Orleans born Bertrand Francois was enlisted into the 2WIR on 25 February 1816, WO25/644. Five members of the 1WIR were killed at the Battle of New Orleans, with a further twenty-three wounded. Return of casualties, 8 January 1815, WO1/141.

[12] Report on 1WIR 1816, WO27/139. On the Bourbon regiment, see Randolph Jones, 'The Bourbon regiment and the Barbados slave revolt of 1816', *Journal of the Society for Army Historical Research* 78 (2000), 3–10.

West Africa had always had a pestilential reputation among the British, similar to that of the West Indies in the eighteenth century, with one resident describing it as 'one of the most unwholesome countries on the face of the earth'.[13] British soldiers sent to Sierra Leone, Gambia or the Gold Coast clearly took a substantial risk, and thus it is not surprising that the Royal African Corps, established in 1800 to garrison these territories, had relied on British soldiers who 'volunteered' for the service after being condemned at a court martial. The rather callous calculation being that as the lives of these men were already forfeit to the state, they might as well serve a brief military purpose. It was not long before a different approach was tried, surely derived from the army's previous experience with the WIRs. Captives liberated from slaving ships after 1807 were usually taken to Sierra Leone, creating a potential pool of new recruits for the army. Between 1808 and 1815 the Royal African Corps was augmented by more than 2,000 liberated Africans who, lacking the language skills to give informed consent, were, as Richard Anderson has pointed out, effectively 'forcibly impressed...on permanent service'.[14] This bi-racial corps was disbanded in 1819, with the 2WIR assuming garrison duties in its place.

Most of the white former soldiers in the Royal African Corps were permitted to settle in South Africa, but more than a hundred were 'considered dangerous' to the peace and security of that colony and so were sent back to West Africa in the early 1820s to form two separate companies attached to the 2WIR.[15] They did not fare well. The outbreak of a 'fever not entirely new but extremely rare' rapidly thinned their ranks. The resident surgeon on the Gold Coast reported, 'There is scarcely one solitary instance of an European arriving here, who is not attacked with the endemic either immediately after his arrival, or within four months'.[16] At Cape Coast Castle the military impact was particularly severe: 'out of the first detachment of European troops that arrived in April 1823...only one survives to tell the

---

[13] Medical topography of Cape Coast, WO334/170. See also Philip Curtin, *The Image of Africa: British Ideas and Action* (Madison: University of Wisconsin Press, 1964), 177–97.

[14] Padraic X. Scanlan, *Freedom's Debtors: British Antislavery in Sierra Leone in the Age of Revolution* (New Haven: Yale University Press, 2017), 118, 125–6; Richard Anderson, 'The diaspora of Sierra Leone's liberated Africans: enlistment, forced migration, and "liberation" at Freetown, 1808–1863', *African Economic History* 41 (2013), 104; *Statistical Report on the Sickness, Mortality and Invaliding among the Troops in Western Africa, St Helena, the Cape of Good Hope and the Mauritius; Prepared from the Records of the Army Medical Department and War-Office Returns* (London: W. Clowes and Sons, 1840), 6.

[15] Goulburn to Merry, 20 November 1821; War Office to Tonens, April 1822, WO43/149.

[16] Medical topography of Cape Coast, WO334/170.

tale', and their wives and children fared no better. Unsurprisingly, the men 'were frequently heard to wish each other a speedy death'.[17] Noting that 'the whole of the black population were exempted from its baneful influence' and cognizant that the health of even the 'most robust' whites who somehow survived had been 'shatter[ed] beyond remedy', army surgeons urged their superiors to 'prevent any more white troops being sent to this pestiferous coast, for so soon as they arrive, so sure will the greatest number of them fall victims to the fever and its destructive consequences'.[18] Their warnings were eventually heeded, and after 1829 the garrison 'consisted entirely of blacks', initially involving detachments from the 1WIR and the 2WIR but augmented in 1840 by 'a native force, at first called the Royal African Corps, now termed the 3rd West India Regiment'.[19] The same military-medical dynamic that had led to the establishment of the WIRs in the 1790s had forced the army's hand in West Africa. Only by transforming the garrisons of West Africa from white to black did the army find a way to tackle an enemy seeking to 'thin the ranks by secret war'.[20]

Although only occasionally involved with active campaigns in the West Indies after 1815, the WIRs continued to prove themselves medically indispensable according to the regimental physicians. When Assistant Staff Surgeon Joseph Allen reported an outbreak of influenza in Demerara (in what is now Guyana) in 1823, 'a very remarkable circumstance occurred in the exemption of the 1st W I regiment from this complaint, for altho' living in the same barracks room with the 21st regiment, they were unmolested by it, as were also the military labourers attached to the garrison'.[21] Seven years later, after a particularly sickly wet season in Demerara when roughly 10 per cent of white troops perished, the garrison surgeon drew an obvious comparison with the 1WIR, which had lost just one man over the same period: 'The efficiency, economy and the health of these black soldiers, in this colony proves to a demonstration, the advantage which would accrue to the Government, under all these heads, were they more extensively employed in the West Indies'.[22] Of course, for all the praise of

[17] Luke Smyth O'Connor, 'Twelve months service in Western Africa', *United Service Journal* (1846), pt 1, 220.

[18] Ibid., 222; Cape Coast and Sierra Leone medical reports 1824, WO334/166 and WO334/170.

[19] *Statistical Report on the Sickness, Mortality and Invaliding among the Troops in Western Africa*, 6; E. J. Burton, 'Observations on the climate, topography, and diseases of the British colonies in Western Africa', *Provincial Medical and Surgical Journal* 3 (1842), 266.

[20] F. Harrison Rankin, *The White Man's Grave: a Visit to Sierra Leone in 1834* (London: Richard Bentley, 1836), II, 167.

[21] Yearly Report 21 Regt Hospital, 20 December 1823, WO334/7.

[22] Observations to accompany the annual return of sick and wounded form the Windward and Leeward Island Command for 1830, WO334/5.

the WIRs from ground commanders, white troops were never going to be fully withdrawn from the West Indies. Island governments and authorities in London wanted the security of at least some white troops in a region that remained heavily reliant on the labour of enslaved Africans.

Such was the expectation that the sickness and mortality rates of black troops would continue to be far lower than European troops, that on the rare occasions when it did not prove to be the case, alarm bells quickly rang in London. When in September 1800 a set of monthly regimental returns arrived on the desk of Secretary at War Henry Dundas, showing higher than normal sickness rates among the WIRs, he immediately wrote to General Thomas Trigge demanding a 'particular explanation. One of the principal inducements for the formation of these corps, was the conviction that they were more competent to all duties of exertion and fatigue and less liable to sickness and the debilitating effects of a tropical climate than European troops, but if these returns are correct, which I confess to you I can scarcely imagine it would lead to a disappointment in one of the chief motives for which they were raised'.[23] Trigge's reply blamed the higher than usual sickness rates on the recent arrival of 'new negroes (by whom alone it is possible to complete these corps)', who were 'equally subject with Europeans to what is termed a seasoning to the climate'. An additional explanation was that most of the black troops had recently been inoculated against smallpox, causing some of them to be 'consequently returned sick'. Trigge stressed that this was a temporary situation and that he fully expected sickness rates to be 'considerably lessened' once the new recruits were 'perfectly seasoned'.[24] The contrast with what had been reported about white soldiers just a few years previously is stark. Seasoning for black soldiers was a short-term inconvenience, whereas for white soldiers the climate was understood to be an 'insuperable bar' to a return to full health, even if the immediate onslaught of disease had been survived. No matter how long white soldiers remained in the West Indies, it was understood that they would never regain their former health, nor match the vitality of their black comrades.[25]

At Prince Rupert's in Dominica the disease environment sometimes became so bad that even members of the WIRs began to suffer. In 1809 it was reported that up to a quarter of the WIR stationed there were 'generally on the sick list'. But once again the situation was far worse for the white garrison, who 'frequently buried 85 men weekly' and spent most of their time digging 'pits in the swamp for patients

[23] Dundas to Trigge, 24 September 1800, WO1/89.
[24] Trigge to Dundas, 20 November 1800, WO1/90.
[25] Army Surgeons to Vaughan, 23 March 1795, WO1/83.

expected to die'.[26] Of course, venturing into the swamp exposed those men to the very mosquitos that spread infections, but the key point to remember is that when placed side by side, in every locale the mortality and sickness rates of WIR soldiers were considerably better than for white troops.

Once Britain's direct involvement with the slave trade ended in 1807, the army's ready supply of Africans was cut off. Fortunately, an alternative appeared almost immediately as the Royal Navy began intercepting ships breaking the slave trade embargo and delivering the liberated slaves to Sierra Leone. An Order in Council issued in 1808 permitted army commanders to select any of these men for the WIRs, and by 1812 a recruiting station had been established in Sierra Leone.[27] Recruits from slave ships were medically problematic. The army's medical director in the West Indies, Robert Jackson, personally attended to the liberated Africans recruited into the WIRs between 1812 and 1815. He thought 'that a small portion of them only were such as I would have selected for soldiers'. Considering that many had been 'plundered' from the coast of Africa, intercepted by the Royal Navy and taken to the Vice-Admiralty Court in Sierra Leone, before being offered to the army, Jackson supposed that after such an ordeal 'they could not be expected to be fit subjects to carry arms', at least not immediately.[28]

The case of the *Regalia* transport ship in 1815 highlighted to a much wider audience the medical issues associated with recruiting men into the WIRs who had been recently liberated from slave ships. The men gathered at Sierra Leone had been 'brought together from various parts of the continent', and many were sick before they even boarded the *Regalia*. About a week into the voyage, Joseph Ollier, the surgeon of the *Porcupine* travelling with the *Regalia*, was summoned to treat the recruits, about fifty of whom were sick 'with ulcer, leprosy and dysentery'. The medical care Ollier was able to offer was extremely limited, partly because each man seemed to speak a different language, and none spoke either English or French.[29] By the time the *Regalia* arrived in Barbados in September

[26] *Grenada Gazette*, 31 December 1836.
[27] *Fourth Report of the Directors of the African Institution* (London: J. Hatchard, 1810), 63–4.
[28] Robert Jackson, *A Sketch of the History and Cure of Febrile Diseases; More Particularly as They Appear in the West Indies among Soldiers of the British Army* (Stockton: T. and H. Eeles, 1817), 591.
[29] Joseph Ollier, Surgeon Officer of the Porcupine to the Transport Board, dated 11 December 1815, in Correspondence of Inspector General William Ferguson, RAMC 212/36 MSS Wellcome Library.

1815, 52 of the 793 recruits had died, and more than 100 went straight to the island's military hospital; a further 70 would perish before the end of the year. William Fergusson, who treated the sick on arrival in Barbados, blamed many of the deaths on 'fluxes', most likely dysentery.[30] The story of the *Regalia* became a matter of public debate. Fergusson published some of the relevant correspondence relating to the *Regalia* case in his study of yellow fever in *Medico Chirurgical Transactions*, and much of it was subsequently reprinted in *The Medical and Physical Journal* the following year. Edward Bancroft's *A Sequel to an Essay on the Yellow Fever* also made extensive use of Fergusson's published report.[31] The *Regalia* was therefore widely discussed and raised important humanitarian issues about the shipment of young African men to the West Indies.[32] Yet the sickly nature of the African recruits was actually not the main focus of most publications that mentioned the *Regalia*. Authors tended to focus on whether the ship had imported yellow fever into the West Indies from Africa, and whether it was even possible to import the disease, given that many believed yellow fever to have local causes related to putrefaction or miasmas. The revelation that WIR recruits were sometimes not in the best of health when they arrived, and were perhaps in general 'much more liable to illness than appears to be generally supposed', did not seem to cause either surprise or alarm. After all, even with the deaths of more than a hundred men from the *Regalia*, nearly 85 per cent were ultimately enlisted into the WIRs. Army commanders were evidently confident that the men from the *Regalia* would eventually be as healthy as other black soldiers in the Caribbean. Neither officials in Whitehall nor army commanders demanded a change in recruitment practices because experience had shown that this was the most effective way of obtaining new soldiers. Even as late as the 1830s, slavers intercepted in West Indian waters provided plenty of new recruits. The Portuguese ship *Negrinha* provided about forty new men for the 1WIR in 1836, while the Spanish

---

[30] William Fergusson, 'An inquiry into the origin and nature of the Yellow Fever', *Medico Chirurgical Transactions* 8 (1817), 109–13; Rana A. Hogarth, *Medicalizing Blackness: Making Racial Difference in the Atlantic World, 1780–1840* (Chapel Hill: University of North Carolina Press, 2017), 71–92. Hogarth concentrates on the issue of immunity to yellow fever in her discussion of the *Regalia*, but I think it unlikely the recruits suffered from yellow fever.

[31] *Medical and Physical Journal* 39 (1818), 149–54; Edward Bancroft, *A Sequel to an Essay on the Yellow Fever* (London: J. Callow, 1817), 217–27.

[32] Wendy D. Churchill, 'Efficient, efficacious and humane responses to non-European bodies in British military medicine, 1780–1815', *The Journal of Imperial and Commonwealth History* 40 (2012), 149–50. One group of liberated slaves in 1843 were described as 'so under size, old, or broken down from hardship they endured on board ship, as to be inadmissible into the service'. O'Connor, 'Twelve months service in western Africa', 217.

registered *Florida* contributed a further sixty.[33] And despite the horrific conditions they had endured during the middle passage, rest combined with a decent diet saw most new arrivals recover their health. As General Thomas Trigge sanguinely put it: 'admitting the utmost that can be allowed, the deaths amongst those people are comparatively small to what the European troops experience'.[34] Thus, in any direct and explicit comparison between the medicalised bodies of European and African soldiers, the latter were usually acknowledged to be superior.

The WIRs were clearly the product of contemporary notions that tropical conditions affected European and African bodies differently, and that Africans were far better equipped to adapt to military service in a hot climate. But once men began to be actually recruited into the regiments, then it was the responsibility of white officers to fashion them into an effective fighting force that could be used to further British imperial aims in the Caribbean. Officers demanded total obedience from their men and thus elevated military discipline above all other characteristics of a soldier. Philip Astley informed the readers of his *Remarks on the Profession and Duty of a Soldier* that 'strict discipline is necessary to the accomplishment of a good soldier' and the only honourable course for a recruit was 'a perfect obedience to the commands of his superior officers'. Anything less would 'lessen the character of a soldier, and ruin the service'.[35] Major Charles James agreed: 'The first principle to be inculcated into the mind of a recruit, is implicit confidence in his captain, and a respectful attention to every commissioned and non-commissioned officer'. He should also be perfectly aware that 'the least deviation will not only expose him to punishment, but prevent his officers from ever granting him the least indulgence'.[36] Could the men of the WIRs be inculcated into military discipline, given that most had been purchased or rescued from slave ships and would have had minimal familiarity with the trappings of military life in a British regiment? A major challenge for

---

[33] *St George's Chronicle*, 1 October 1836; *Port of Spain Gazette*, 19 May 1837. A number of these new African recruits subsequently mutinied, see Thomas August, 'Rebels with a cause: the St Joseph mutiny of 1837', *Slavery and Abolition* 12 (1991), 73–91. *HMS Vestal* brought another group of liberated Africans into Grenada, resulting in 112 'able-bodied and clean-limbed recruits' for 1WIR. Luke Smyth O'Connor, 'Suggestions for the discipline, uniform, messing and recruiting of the West India regiments', *United Service Journal* (1837), pt 1, 364.

[34] Trigge to Dundas, 20 November 1800, WO1/90. Mortality rates in 1817 were 16.2 per cent for white troops, but only 4.6 per cent for black troops. *Statistical Reports for the West Indies*, 5, 11.

[35] Philip Astley, *Remarks on the Profession and Duty of a Soldier* (London: for the author, 1794), 11–12.

[36] Charles James, *The Regimental Companion* (London: T. Egerton, 1800), I, 302–3.

white officers of the WIRs trying to enforce obedience was how to convey what was expected in the first place among recruits whose grasp of English ranged from limited to non-existent.

Bi-annual inspection reports filed by senior officers provide an insight into how WIR soldiers were perceived by their commanders. In an era when attitudes toward non-white people were both shaped and then reinforced by the institution of slavery, one might expect that WIR commanders would have a largely negative view of these mainly African-born recruits. Indeed, Lieutenant Colonel John Lyons Nixon, commanding in Antigua, was somewhat underwhelmed by the NCOs of the 4WIR, declaring that they were 'for the most part very stupid they have not the least notion of supporting their authority over their men as Europeans would tho' the greatest pains have been taken to include this principle into their minds'. Lieutenant Colonel Clement William Whitby of the 1WIR was similarly critical of 'the great want of intelligence on the part of the black NCOs' that meant they were 'not so very useful as might otherwise be the case'. General George Don, inspecting the 4WIR on its arrival in Gibraltar in 1817, grumbled that 'the non-commissioned officers and privates of this corps are in general a weakly class of men and do not seem to possess the physical powers or intellect of Europeans'. Yet these views were actually out of step with the vast majority of those who inspected the WIRs on a regular basis. Most of the time black sergeants and corporals were described as 'active', 'intelligent', 'obedient', 'respectful', 'attentive' and 'willing', all ideal qualities that any commander would value. These judgements were inevitably subjective, and the commander of the 5WIR in Jamaica acknowledged that the black NCOs 'are carefully selected from amongst the most intelligent and well conducted men of the corps, ... as far as the capacity of men of the class they are of will allow'. The lower intellectual capacity of black soldiers was a given: no one expected black NCOs to match the most capable of their white counterparts, only that they would 'act to the best of their limited abilities'. Despite this, even those critical of the intelligence of WIR soldiers thought they had redeeming features. Lieutenant Colonel Nixon might have believed his NCOs to be 'very stupid', but they were also 'very obedient and respectful to their officers ... willing and well disposed', while their 'naturally very violent' tendencies were a positive plus. General Don observed that the men of the 4WIR in Gibraltar were 'quiet and well-disposed and conduct themselves properly', while Lieutenant Colonel Whitby grudgingly admitted that when 'considerable pains are taken to give them practical instruction; as long as they retain it, they get on fixedly well'.[37]

---

[37] Reports for the 4WIR 1815, 1WIR 1819, 4WIR 1817, 3WIR 1812, 5WIR 1815, 4WIR 1812 and 1WIR 1816, WO27/113, 133, 139, 141, 147.

Perceptions of rank-and-file soldiers were generally similar to those of NCOs. The vast majority of inspection reports described the men as 'good', or 'very good' or even 'a fine body of men' who 'surpassed my most sanguine expectations' and were, perhaps in contrast to some other regiments, 'extremely clean'. The commander of the 1WIR in Barbados thought it noteworthy that 'they bathe in the sea every Saturday morning'.[38] Thomas Hislop in Demerara constantly found newly arrived Africans preferable to local recruits since 'I have invariably found them to make the most orderly, clean and attentive soldiers'.[39] The linguistic barriers were inevitably considerable: 'Great difficulty attends their drilling and instruction as one half do not speak English'. Their performance despite this hindrance was generally praised: 'The march in line is steady and correct, and considering that they scarcely understand a word of any known language their performance is wonderful'. Just occasionally, a commander would complain that 'from the pains which are taken to drill them, a much more military air ought to exist than is observable; they want military feelings and pride', yet such sentiments were definitely not the norm. The commander of the 2WIR believed his men had 'a great esprit du corps', while Major General John Montagu Mainwaring described the 1WIR as 'extremely well disciplined' and awarded them perhaps the ultimate accolade: 'soldierlike'. It is perhaps significant that Mainwaring, before assuming command of the 1WIR had captained a troop of Black Dragoons in Grenada in the 1790s.[40]

There was general agreement, therefore, that WIR soldiers were obedient, diligent and committed, but there was also a growing recognition of their military utility. While some may have considered the WIRs ideal for nothing more than garrison duty in insalubrious locales, they were quickly thrust into active campaigning. Observing a newly embodied regiment in Barbados in 1796, George Pinckard described them as 'active and expert' and believed that they had the making of a 'formidable corps'.[41] Those leading the regiments in battle often described

---

[38] Report for the 1WIR, WO27/147.

[39] 'Hislop's remarks on the establishment of West India regiments written in the year 1801', 6 WO1/95.

[40] The commander of the 1WIR in Trinidad in 1809 also described them as 'soldierlike'. Charles R. Dodd, *The Annual Biography* (London: Chapman and Hall, 1843), 420. Reports for 1WIR 1809, 6WIR 1812, 1WIR 1812, 7WIR 1815, 1WIR 1819, 5WIR 1812, 2WIR 1817, 1WIR 1819, 2WIR 1817 and 1WIR 1820 and 1822, WO27/97, 113, 133, 139, 141, 147, 149, 155.

[41] George Pinckard, *Notes on the West Indies* (London: Baldwin, Cradock and Joy, 1816), I, 208.

them in glowing terms. General John Moore, commanding in St Lucia in 1796, thought they 'possess[ed] ... many excellent qualities as soldiers, and may with proper attention become equal to anything'.[42] Moore compared the WIR troops under his command favourably with the white regiments serving alongside them. The 'total want of discipline and interior economy' among white regiments could be solved, he thought, by a little more bathing and sobriety for which the WIR were renowned.[43] Thomas Hislop who formed the South American Rangers in Demerara, later embodied as the 11WIR, was just as enthusiastic about black soldiers: 'The utility of them, has in every instance been fully proved, whether by their services in the field or by their capability of performing every other description of military duties'.[44]

Even before the regiments were formally constituted, those fighting in the Caribbean were deeply impressed by the martial qualities of black soldiers. Colonel Robert Brisbane, commanding an informal black corps in St Domingue in 1794, thought they showed 'uncommon bravery' and reported: 'I have been eye witness to the merits of a black corps and am of opinion that they are the only people to employ upon all occasions ... the mulattoes dread nothing so much as to fight against Negroes'.[45] The following year the commanding officer in Dominica reported to his superiors that 'the coloured compy headed by Mr Johnston conducted themselves like heroes' during a battle near Roseau. 'I do not think I ever saw men so anxious to advance or do it with more alertness or spirit'.[46] In January 1795 the remnants of the Carolina Corps were dispatched to St Lucia to deal with the 'revolted Negroes'. Although the attack was unsuccessful, General Sir John Vaughan praised the 'great bravery' and 'great spirit' of the men. A few months later he informed the War Office that 'it is to the Black corps under Lieut Colonel Soter that we owe the possession of Martinicio at this moment. It is to the lately raised Corps of Blacks under Capt Malcolm that we have been able to retain our footing in St Lucia. I do aver, that had it not been for the services of these two provincial corps that both these islands would before now have been lost'. Such was the martial prowess of black troops that every time they

[42] Add MSS 57327 Sir John Moore Papers, 5v British Library.
[43] J. F. Maurice, *The Diary of Sir John Moore* (London: Edward Arnold, 1904), 236; see also Catherine Kelly, *War and the Militarization of British Army Medicine, 1793–1830* (London: Pickering and Chatto, 2011), 27–9.
[44] Roger N. Buckley (ed.), 'Brigadier-General Thomas Hislop's remarks on the establishment of the West India Regiments – 1801', *Journal of the Society for Army Historical Research* 58 (1980), 210; 'Hislop's Remarks', WO1/95.
[45] Brisbane to Williamson, 20 and 24 September 1794, WO1/60.
[46] Bagot to Vaughan, 14 June 1795, WO1/31.

had been sent into difficult terrain against rebel slaves, they distinguished themselves by their 'intrepidity and alacrity'.[47]

As the war in West Indies dragged on into the new century, and the British strove to cling to the islands they had wrested from the French, the WIRs proved their military worth again and again and were mentioned in dispatches on numerous occasions. In 1801 Sir Thomas Trigge was fulsome in his praise of the 8WIR during the capture of St Maarten. They had 'evinced the greatest courage and steadiness: they repulsed and pursued the enemy, and took possession of the two field pieces... that a regiment like the 8th, formed within the last three years, and composed almost entirely of new negroes, who never before had seen an enemy, should engage with the gallantry they did, and behave in a manner that would do honor to any troops'. During a naval assault on Marie Galante that same year, the commander of three companies from the 1WIR took 'great pleasure in making known to the army his entire approbation of the spirit manifested by this detachment'.[48]

News of the exceptional bravery of the WIRs seeped slowly into the public domain. During the conquest of Martinique in April 1809, it was widely reported that 'none were more brave or active than the flank companies of the 3rd West India Regt and 8th'. The assault on Fort Bourbon in Martinique, one of the strongest fortresses in the West Indies, was singled out more than once as a time when WIR soldiers displayed 'European courage'.[49] Several of the WIRs earned battle honours for their achievements in Dominica, Martinique and Guadeloupe. Dispatches from army commanders praising 'the gallant conduct of the black troops at the attack of Martinique' were printed in British newspapers and commented on in Parliament. MP James Stephen was surely not the only one who noticed that the WIRs were 'extolled by almost every General under whom they were engaged in active service'.[50] When a plan was mooted to transplant the WIRs to India, one of

[47] Vaughan to Dundas, 31 January 1795, 25 February 1795, 16 April 1795, WO1/83; 'Hislop's Remarks', 2 WO1/95.

[48] Report on the West India regiments, 56, 60 CO320/3.

[49] Prevost to Meyers, 1 March 1805, cited in Thomas Southey, *Chronological History of the West Indies* (London: Longman, 1827) v.3, 312. General orders 9, September 1808, WO1/96; Fergusson, *Notes and Recollections of a Professional Life*, 208.

[50] Local newspapers reprinted the *London Gazette*'s account – *Chester Courant*, 6 June 1809, *Kentish Gazette*, 9 June 1809. *Cobbett's Parliamentary Debates* (London: Hansard, 1809), v.14, 898. Stephen had spent time on St Kitts, supplying his brother-in-law William Wilberforce with inside information on West Indian slavery. For a biography of Stephens, see www.historyofparliamentonline.org/volume/1790-1820/member/stephen-james-1758-1832; Stephen, *Slavery in the British West India Colonies Delineated*, I, 427. These commendations for bravery were still being remarked upon thirty years later. See *Antigua Messenger*, 29 December 1836, and *St George's Chronicle and Grenada Gazette*, 25 March 1837.

the arguments used in support was that their 'personal strength and courage are generally estimated superior to the natives of Hindostan'.[51] The 'great gallantry' of the WIRs even attracted international attention with the Boston *Columbian Centinel* reporting in 1805 that during a recent action in Dominica black troops 'shared the laurels', and that 'it is owing to them in an eminent degree, that the British flag now flies at Dominica'.[52]

Some attributed the martial skills of the WIRs to a careful policy of purchasing the right sorts of Africans to be soldiers. Those tasked with obtaining new recruits for the WIRs were instructed to pay particular attention to the ethnic origin of the men. Just as Africans from particular regions were valued by slaveholders due to their supposed docility or physical prowess, certain other ethnic groups had reputations as being more ferocious or having a martial tradition. In 1798, after a delivery for the 8WIR of 'poor puny looking men' mainly from Angola, Dominica Governor Andrew James Cochrane-Johnstone declared that he would 'have none but Ebos and Coromantees and Creoles'. Writing to Secretary of War Henry Dundas, he 'strongly recommended ... that the negroes for the other black corps should be all composed if possible of the Coromanty race, who are a warlike nation and particularly fond of fire arms'.[53] Johnstone's views concorded with contemporary ideas of the 'national character' of Africans circulating among white West Indians. For Edward Long, the widely read historian of Jamaica, 'Coromantin Negroes ... are distinguished from their brethren by their aversion to husbandry, and the martial ferocity of their disposition'.[54] Bryan Edwards agreed: 'the circumstances which distinguish the Koromantyn, or Gold Coast, Negroes, from all others, are firmness both of body and mind; and ferociousness of disposition ... which prompts them to enterprizes of difficulty and danger; and enables them to meet death, in its most horrible shape, with fortitude or indifference'.[55] These people were almost certainly Asante people from what is now Ghana, and their involvement in numerous slave revolts in Jamaica seemingly confirmed their general unsuitability for slavery but made them ideal recruits into the WIRs. Thomas Hislop urged recruiters for the WIRs to seek out those 'who, in their own country are habituated to the dangers and hardships of a soldier's life', and in particular recommended 'the

---

[51] IOR MSS EU E293/134 British Library.

[52] *Columbian Centinel*, 24 July 1805.

[53] Cochrane to Dundas, 7 June 1798, WO1/88.

[54] Edward Long, *History of Jamaica* (London: John Stockdale, 1774), II, 446.

[55] Bryan Edwards, *History, Civil and Commercial, of the British Colonies in the West Indies* (London: John Stockdale, 1793), II, 63.

Coromantees [who] are reckoned amongst the most intrepid and hardy, being trained from their infancy to war. The Fantees and Angolas are also esteemed a spirited and an active race of people'.[56] Unfortunately most of the early succession books for the WIRs have been lost, so a comprehensive and detailed analysis of the ethnic origins of purchased men is impossible. Data from the 5WIR suggests that the Coromantee actually only formed a very small percentage of recruits, with Eboes from the Bight of Biafra and those from Congo forming the two largest ethnic groups.[57]

Within a few years of the establishment of the WIRs, commanders had come to the broad conclusion that these men were highly capable soldiers, with exactly the sort of spirit they were looking for. The question now became whether these men had the physical robustness to sustain their position as soldiers par excellence. It was, of course, already widely accepted and understood that black troops were highly resistant to tropical diseases, and the regular returns from the regiments confirmed as much, but what about the day-to-day exertions required of a soldier? The job of maintaining military bodies lay with regimental surgeons and their assistants who dealt with every kind of injury and ailment. These men had just one responsibility: to provide medical care to the soldiers so that the army had sufficient fit and healthy troops when they were needed. Maintaining the regiment as a viable fighting force was naturally the highest priority for commanders in chief, and therefore all surgeons were supposed to maintain a complete and accurate record of every case they treated, including medicines used and the eventual outcome. Statistics as to the fitness of the regiment were reported on a monthly basis by regimental commanding officers to the War Office. The men of the WIRs turned out to be a source of constant fascination for white regimental surgeons in the early nineteenth century. Few of those posted to serve in the Caribbean would have had extensive prior experience of treating those of African descent, indeed many were fresh from Scottish medical schools.[58] Their new posting would involve interpreting and reinterpreting black bodies, as well as determining and navigating perceived differences with white bodies.

---

[56] 'Hislop's Remarks', 7–8 WO1/95.

[57] Roger Norman Buckley, *Slaves in Red Coats: the British West India Regiments, 1795–1815* (New Haven: Yale University Press, 1979), 115. As Buckley notes, data on origins is imprecise, since it might refer to place of embarkation rather than birth.

[58] As late as the 1840s, 86 per cent of army surgeons had a Scottish medical qualification. Spencer H. Brown, 'British army surgeons commissioned 1840–1909 with West Indian/West African service: a prosopographical evaluation', *Medical History* 37 (1993), 422.

Several historians have pointed to the transformation of British military medicine that was driven by experiences in the West Indies, indeed Mark Harrison has argued convincingly that 'by far the most important centres of medical activity in the East and West Indies were the medical establishments of the armed forces'.[59] Military doctors in the eighteenth century were the first to stress the importance of allowing for the seasoning of newly arrived British troops, and the hundreds of medical personal who served in the Caribbean helped to develop 'a distinct empirical and experimental approach to medicine particular to the tropics', one that 'favoured observation and experiment'.[60] Many of these physicians were attached to white regiments that were posted to the West Indies for a period of years, and as such had minimal contact with WIR troops. But between the founding of the WIRs in 1795 through the consolidation of the force into just two regiments in 1825, nearly a hundred surgeons were either directly attached to the WIRs or posted to garrison hospitals that treated all medical cases on a particular island. Surgeons officially attached to the WIRs served with them, on average, for more than two years and some for much longer. Thomas Murray joined the 5WIR in 1805, transferred to the 2WIR in 1811 and finally retired in 1820. Collin Allan was appointed as assistant surgeon for the 7WIR in 1803, promoted to surgeon in 1806 and remained with the regiment, mainly serving in Honduras, until it was disbanded in 1816.[61] Murray, Allan and those like them had the time to become deeply familiar with the men of the regiment. They would have known which individuals had long-standing medical conditions, those who were most frequently sick and those who never troubled them. If they had previously served with a white regiment, or if they spent time in the garrison hospital, they would have been able to draw explicit comparisons between the ailments that afflicted European and African soldiers.

Surgeons had played a crucial role in the creation of the regiments in the 1790s. Once it became apparent that West Indian plantations were

---

[59] Mark Harrison, *Medicine in an Age of Commerce and Empire: Britain and Its Tropical Colonies, 1660–1830* (Oxford: Oxford University Press, 2010).

[60] Suman Seth, *Difference and Disease: Medicine, Race and the Eighteenth-Century British Empire* (Cambridge: Cambridge University Press, 2018), 94. Kelly, *War and the Militarization of British Army Medicine*, 11, 27. See also J. D. Alsop, 'Warfare and the creation of British imperial medicine, 1600–1800', in G. Hudson (ed.), *British Military and Naval Medicine, 1600–1830* (Amsterdam: Rodopi, 2007), 23–50.

[61] *Commissioned Officers in the Medical Service of the British Army, 1660–1960* (London: Wellcome Historical Medical Library, 1968), 165, 93. Succession book of the 7WIR, WO25/660. As the disease environment for whites improved in the second half of the nineteenth century, the average length of service for surgeons posted to tropical locations increased to eighteen years. Brown, 'British army surgeons', 425.

never going to supply sufficient men for the army, the decision was taken to concentrate on purchasing men from slave ships. Specific instructions were given in 1797 to army selectors: men should be between eighteen and thirty years of age, at least 5'5" high and 'of a sound body'. Furthermore, two 'principal medical staff' would examine and approve each recruit.[62] This process established a 'norm' for black bodies in the minds of regimental surgeons. Aware that the middle passage took a toll on the health of those forced to endure it, and concerned that unsuitable enslaved men would be palmed off on the army by unscrupulous traders, medical staff took particular pains to check the age of the recruits 'as the age of a negro is not easily known', including taking advice from 'some good judges' more used to inspecting enslaved bodies.[63] A year later the guidelines had been relaxed a little, recruits just 16 years old would be accepted and 'growing boys' of 5'3" would pass inspection, but the army remained adamant that every man purchased 'shall not be deformed, maimed, or injured in any respect, but stout, able-bodied, healthy men, capable of bearing arms'.[64]

Some of the men successfully recruited for the WIRs were indeed 'well sized and proportioned'. Major General Edward Stehelin described the men of the 3WIR in Barbados in 1812 as a 'good, stout body of men, most from five feet five to five feet nine inches, a few over, and not many under, with a general appearance of health'.[65] Other regiments were not so fortunate, and the recruiting station that operated in Sierra Leone between 1812 and 1816 was especially indiscriminate. A group of recruits who arrived in Martinique in 1814 for the 4WIR included Joseph Richards, age nine, as well as four others ages ten and eleven.[66] Of course those recording ages were almost certainly guessing, based on height, whether the recruit had gone through puberty, and perhaps the number of adult teeth. The recruits themselves would have been unable to convey the necessary information in a European language. Even adult recruits sometimes failed to meet the supposed height requirement. The inspector of the 7WIR in Curacao in 1812 reported 'many low' men, while the 3WIR in Trinidad in 1815 contained men 'low in stature...many boys and some very small'. Just 46 per cent of the 4WIR were over 5'5" tall when inspected in 1817. By contrast, in two white regiments stationed

---

[62] Instructions to Hunter, 26 January 1797, WO1/86.
[63] Instructions for the officers and medical staff, WO1/86.
[64] Contact with Samuel Chollet 19 March 1798, Instructions to Lt. Col. Booth, WO1/86.
[65] 1WIR 1809, WO27/97; 3WIR 1812, WO27/113.
[66] 4WIR succession book, WO25/653. Anderson, 'The diaspora of Sierra Leone's liberated Africans', 106–8.

alongside the 4WIR, 72 per cent and 85 per cent of rank-and-file soldiers were over 5'5".[67] The situation improved considerably with the reduction in the number of WIRs after 1815. The fittest men were drafted into the remaining regiments and by 1820 only 8 per cent of the men in the 1WIR were under 5'5".[68]

Despite their often-diminutive stature, commanding officers and surgeons began to notice physically impressive traits among WIR soldiers that built on and expanded earlier tropes about black bodies. George Pinckard served as a medical officer with General Sir Ralph Abercromby's expedition against St Domingue in 1796–7. Amidst his generally gloomy observations on the disastrous campaign, he noted the rapid recovery of wounded black soldiers compared to their white counterparts: 'The distress occasioned by [wounds and ulcers] is wholly confined to the Europeans; for, while the soldiers from England continue to suffer dreadfully from their sores, the wounds of the Africans, who are lying in the adjoining beds of the same wards, heal with surprising rapidity, and are completely cured. Indeed the recovery from sores and ulcers in this climate is as peculiarly successful among the blacks, as it is the reverse among the Europeans'.[69] Leonard Gillespie, a surgeon at the main military hospital on Martinique, observed the same phenomenon among his patients who had been wounded on campaign in St Lucia in early 1796. Many of the injured white soldiers died of gangrenous wounds, something he attributed to 'the unhealthy, moist, calm and sultry state of the weather'. The wounds of the black soldiers, however, 'were much less exposed to this change than the whites: left in some measure to dress their own sores, and habituated to the climate, they recovered'. Based on this observation, Gillespie decided not to amputate the legs of two black soldiers who had received bad knee wounds but instead let them recover naturally. Although the joints were 'achilosed' or fused, and therefore no longer flexible, the experiment had proved that for black soldiers at least 'amputation is not ever indispensably necessary'.[70] Moreover, some believed that rapid healing and recovery from injury was not only the preserve of black soldiers, it applied to all those of African descent. George Pinckard narrated the story of a plantation

---

[67] 7WIR Curacao 1812, WO27/113; 3WIR Trinidad 1815, WO27/133; Muster book of the 4WIR, WO25/653; Inspection Reports 1817 for 4WIR, 11th and 60th regiments, all stationed in Gibraltar, WO27/141.

[68] Report for 1WIR, WO27/149.

[69] Pinckard, *Notes on the West Indies*, II, 134–5.

[70] Leonard Gillespie, *Observations on the Diseases Which Prevailed on Board a Part of His Majesty's Squadron on the Leeward Island Station between November 1794 and April 1796* (London: G. Auld, 1800), 17.

slave who was severely wounded in the head by a cutlass and 'one of the blows, passed through the bones of the scull and the membranes, into the substance of the brain'. Despite such a traumatic injury, 'the negro rapidly recovered, and is now alive and well'.[71]

The healing powers of black soldiers thus began to enter the medical literature as an established fact, reinforcing other ideas about the robust nature of the black body, and it continued a trend of army physicians publicising what they thought were key medical differences between white and black people. Benjamin Moseley, surgeon general of Jamaica in the 1760s and 1770s, made a number of observations about physical differences between those of European and African descent. African women, for instance, 'soon recover from lying-in; ... often mak[ing] it an affair of a few days, and sometimes of a few hours only, and then pursue their occupation'.[72] Edward Long had made a very similar observation in 1774: 'their women are delivered with little or no labour ... some have even been known to bring forth twins without a shriek, or a scream; and it is seldom they are confined above two, or, at most, three days'.[73] When Moseley joined the Nicaraguan campaign of 1781 that included white regiments and large numbers of black pioneers, he reported that black people 'bear chirurgical operations much better than white people and what would be the cause of insupportable pain to a white man, a Negro would almost disregard. I have amputated the legs of many Negroes, who have held the upper part of the limb themselves'.[74] The importance of Moseley and Pinckard in particular lies in the wide readership of their publications. Moseley's book quickly became a standard text for those interested in tropical medicine and went through at least four revised editions between 1787 and 1803. His claim that black people were insensible to pain was still being cited in numerous texts more than sixty years later.[75] Pinckard's colourful vignettes of life in the

---

[71] Pinckard, *Notes on the West Indies*, II, 135–6.

[72] Benjamin Moseley, *A Treatise on Tropical Diseases on Military Operations* (London: T. Cadell, 1787), 61. See also Martin S. Pernick, *A Calculus of Suffering: Pain, Professionalism, and Anesthesia in Nineteenth-Century America* (New York: Columbia University Press, 1985), 148–60.

[73] Long, *History of Jamaica*, II, 380.

[74] Moseley, *A Treatise on Tropical Diseases*, 475.

[75] See, for example, *Transactions of the American Philosophical Society*, 4 (1799), 292; *The Monthly Magazine, and American Review*, 2 (1800), 299; William Frederick Van Amringe, *An investigation of the Theories of the Natural History of Man* (New York: Baker and Scribner, 1848), 392; Josiah Priest, *Slavery, as It Relates to the Negro, or African Race* (Louisville: W. S. Brown, 1849), 241; Joseph A. Gobineau (Josiah Nott trans.), *The Moral and Intellectual Diversity of Races* (Philadelphia: J. Lippincott, 1856), 447; John Campbell, *Negro-Mania: Being an Examination of the Falsely Assumed Equality of the Various Races of Men* (Philadelphia: Campbell and Power, 1851), 133. See also Seth, *Difference and Disease*, 153.

West Indies attracted those of a less scientific frame of mind, but the original edition of 1806 was still popular enough to be expanded for a second edition in 1816.

The ability to withstand pain, and to heal quickly, was attributed by several physicians to Africans having thicker skin than Europeans. Dr Charles White, writing in 1799, thought 'the skin, including the epidermis and rete muscosum, is well known to be thicker in the African than in the Europeans'.[76] It was this same attribute that meant 'he is much better adapted to bear the effects of extreme heat and exposure to the solar rays of a tropical climate than Europeans are'. Indeed, one army surgeon believed that such was the 'greater density and toughness' of this layer of skin that it was 'often sufficient to turn the front of a lancet'.[77] William Fergusson remarked, 'One of the most obvious peculiarities of the Negro, compared with the European, is the texture of his skin, which is thick, oily, and rank'. Importantly, however, he suggested that this thicker skin helped to prevent 'marsh poison' (the supposed cause of tropical fevers) from infecting black people as easily as it did whites.[78] Reporting on a yellow fever epidemic in Guiana that had seen a 13 per cent white mortality rate but less than 1 per cent among black inhabitants, Daniel Blair believed the data confirmed 'the importance of the skin' in protecting those of African descent.[79] Possession of this particularly tough skin was of immense importance for a soldier. Effectively it functioned as a type of natural armour, protecting the owner from harm, and it left the white soldier, by contrast, seeming rather fragile with his easily damaged skin, leaving him acutely vulnerable to the worst that West Indian service could throw at him.

The supposed outer toughness of black skin was often used as a justification for the harsh physical punishments meted out to enslaved people in the Americas, and the records of regimental courts martial demonstrate that the soldiers of the WIRs were victims of the same racist stereotyping. Each regiment was required to submit a list of regimental courts martial with their bi-annual inspection return. The form contains information on offenders, what they were charged with and if convicted what the punishment was. Punishments of NCOs and privates essentially took

[76] Charles White, *An Account of the Regular Gradation in Man* (London: C. Dilly, 1799), 57. Here I diverge from Wendy Churchill's assertion that positive medical traits among non-whites were 'interpreted as features of their barbarism'. Churchill, 'Efficient, efficacious and humane responses', 141.

[77] Reports into delirium tremens 9 March 1841, Return of 2nd WIR in Bahamas, WO334/174.

[78] Fergusson, *Notes and Recollections of a Professional Life*, 203.

[79] Daniel Blair, *Report on the First Eighteen Months of the Fourth Yellow Fever Epidemic of British Guiana* (pamphlet 1856), 80.

four forms: lashes, solitary confinement for a fixed period, stoppages of pay and, if an officer, a reduction of rank. Crucially, records list the initial sentence together with the punishment actually carried out. When a soldier was to receive lashes, 'a disagreeable duty devolves on the surgeon; for no man by the military laws, can be flogged without his attendance. It becomes his business diligently to watch over the sufferers; for should the punishment adjudged prove greater than it is his opinion the delinquent can bear without hazard of his life, he has authority to stop the Drummers (the executioners) at any period of it, and order him to be taken down'.[80] The regimental surgeon therefore was required to make a judgement call on each individual's capacity to withstand physical pain and how their body would respond. It was his responsibility 'to ascertain *the extreme limit of human endurance*'.[81] Commanding officers did not always take note of the surgeon's recommendation. Henry Marshall recounted the tale of one poor man in the West Indies who was sentenced to 500 lashes; when the surgeon tried to intervene after 250 lashes, the commander had the surgeon imprisoned for ten days for interference.[82] In general, however, the army had no intention of wasting the effort and resources it had invested in a soldier by beating him to death.

Robert Hamilton, whose *Duties of a Regimental surgeon* went through several editions from 1787 on, gave detailed advice on how a flogging should be administered. The target area should be the well-muscled shoulders, not the lower back where damage might be done to the ribs or vital organs. He recommended against stopping a punishment only to continue it at a later date since the damage to partially healed skin would be worse than if the flogging had just continued to its conclusion. Above all, he believed it to be the surgeon's duty to understand 'the form of the sufferer's body; the make of his fibre, and the strength of his constitution'. While individuals would inevitably respond differently to a flogging, with small slight men faring worse than tall, heavily set men, Hamilton also highlighted the importance of different types of skin. He argued that 'those … of a dark, or brown complexion … are generally of a robust constitution' and these men 'are always stronger and abler to bear punishment'.[83] Soldiers of the WIRs had the blackest skin of any men in the army, and therefore by this logic were able to withstand greater punishment than European soldiers.

[80]   Robert Hamilton, *The Duties of a Regimental Surgeon Considered* (London: J. Johnson, 1787), II, 27.
[81]   Henry Marshall, *Military Miscellany* (London: John Murray, 1846), 276.
[82]   Henry Marshall, 'A historical sketch of military punishments, in as far as regards non-commissioned officers and private soldiers', *United Service Journal* (1844), pt 2, 255.
[83]   Ibid., 48–9.

Although some white men joined the WIRs in the very earliest years, the courts martial records do not survive to tell us if they were treated more leniently than black men. White sergeants, who served with the WIRs throughout their existence, proved problematic for regimental commanders. Often extra license was granted to them precisely because of 'the inconvenience of reducing them to the ranks'.[84] The two years the 4WIR spent in Gibraltar actually provides the best test case for examining the differing application of punishments to regular black and white soldiers. When based in the West Indies the WIRs usually occupied isolated posts some distance from white regiments, but in Gibraltar the 4WIR was in close proximity to the white regiments also stationed there. Comparing the regimental returns from the 4WIR with those of the 11th, 26th, 60th and 64th regiments between 1817 and 1819 reveals a clear racialised difference in the way military discipline operated. Soldiers of the 4WIR were twice as likely to be court-martialled than white soldiers of the 11th regiment who shared the Casemates Barracks, and more than half of those convicted (54.5 per cent) received lashes. Only 27.4 per cent of white soldiers convicted in courts martial in Gibraltar received lashes. In some locations physical punishment was the only option since 'black holes, and places for solitary confinement, properly constructed, are not established'.[85] But prevalent racist ideas also clearly had an impact on the different types of punishment meted out on white and black bodies. One officer believed in 'the necessity of a certain degree of severity' for black troops since 'solitary confinement is no punishment to men whose greatest enjoyment comes in idleness'. Leniency would perhaps 'be attended with dangerous consequences'.[86] These same ideas ensured that fugitive slaves held in jails before being claimed by owners were required to undertake physical exercise, sometimes on treadmills.[87] The isolation and mental inactivity of confinement was evidently deemed punishment enough for many white men.

Not only were white soldiers beaten less frequently than black soldiers, they were also much more likely to receive a reduction in their original number of lashes. On aggregate, 61 per cent of the lashes awarded were actually inflicted on WIR soldiers. The corresponding figures for white regiments in Gibraltar were 36 per cent, 42 per cent, 41 per cent and

---

[84] York to Liverpool, 15 August 1811, WO1/647.
[85] Report of 5WIR 1812, WO27/108.
[86] Report of 6WIR 1812, WO27/113. See also the Report for the 7WIR 1806, WO27/90, where the inspector commented there had been 'great necessity' for 'very numerous' courts martial.
[87] See, for example, Barry W. Higman, *Slave Populations of the British Caribbean 1807–1834* (Kingston: University of the West Indies Press, 1995), 243; and Randy M. Browne, *Surviving Slavery in the British Caribbean* (Philadelphia: University of Pennsylvania Press, 2017), 54.

39 per cent. Surgeons supervising these lashings therefore intervened on average before white soldiers had received half their allotted number of stripes. Black soldiers endured about 50 per cent more lashes and this can only be because regimental surgeons had accepted Hamilton's understanding of the different nature of black and white skin.[88] A belief in the physical robustness of WIR soldiers clearly had some highly negative consequences, but a few officers also questioned the efficacy of beatings for black troops thinking, perhaps, that the thicker skin of black troops was so tough that beating was not much of a punishment at all. One old officer recommended other punishments such as 'turning the coat', that marked out malefactors for ridicule from their peers, would be more effective at reforming those 'who had appeared irreclaimable'.[89] Colonel Lyle Carmichael, commanding the 2WIR, used the men's pride in their uniform and soldierly accoutrements. He was convinced that 'degrading otherwise incorrigible offenders, depriving them of their arms and appointments and not permitting them any except fatigue duties had frequently an effect where punishment of another nature fail'd'.[90]

The army was fairly set in its ways, however, and tended to rely on corporeal punishment. The data for the 4WIR in Gibraltar largely concords with data for other WIRs in the West Indies. A sample of returns between 1812 and 1825 proves that WIR soldiers received, on average, 69 per cent of the lashes awarded. Before the maximum sentence was limited at 300 lashes in 1812, some WIR soldiers were sentenced to as many as 999 lashes. The maximum number inflicted, according to surviving records was 600 meted out to Private Joseph of the 1WIR in 1812 for stealing, gambling and striking two superior officers. Despite the high level of physical chastisement, however, some regimental surgeons believed that 'compared to slavery the restrictions of military discipline are an exquisite freedom'.[91] And when the diaries of West Indian planters such

---

[88]   Studies of other white regiments confirms that only about half of convicted white soldiers received the full sentence. G. A. Steppler, 'British military law, discipline, and the conduct of regimental courts martial in the later eighteenth century', *The English Historical Review* 102 (1987), 877.

[89]   *Letter of an Old Field Officer on Military Punishments* (London: The author, 1837), 20.

[90]   Carmichael to Castlereagh, 10 September 1808, CO137/123.

[91]   The order from the commander in chief limiting the number of lashes to 300 was dated 25 March 1812, and is reprinted in Marshall, *Military Miscellany*, 184–5. The oft cited date is 1829, but that refers to the change in the law. Peter Burroughs, 'Crime and punishment in the British Army, 1815–1870', *English Historical Review* 100 (1985), 562; 1WIR WO27/113; Pinckard, *Notes on the West Indies*, II, 130. The largest number of lashes ever ordered by a court martial was 1500, given to a solider of the 67th regiment serving in Bengal in 1807. Henry Marshall, 'A historical sketch of military punishments', *United Service Journal* (1843), pt 3, 109.

Thomas Thistlewood are replete with examples of far more gruesome tortures inflected on black bodies, perhaps they were right.[92]

Regimental surgeons who worked with black soldiers on a daily basis began to notice other interesting divergences between white troops and the soldiers of the WIRs. Considering that 'in no part of the world is sexual intercourse more general or carried to greater excess than amongst the black population. It is a remarkable circumstance', wrote one regimental surgeon, that black soldiers seemed to be 'exempt from abrasion and excoriation which happen to white soldiers'.[93] The supposed tough skin of black men was, some thought, even capable of deflecting sexually transmitted diseases. Aside from thicker skin, the surgeon attached to the 2WIR, John Richardson, observed the singular immunity of his soldiers to 'delirium tremens' or the withdrawal symptoms suffered by alcoholics. Indeed, there was general agreement that 'the blacks possessed also an invaluable superiority over the white troops, in their sobriety'.[94] One correspondent of the *United Service Journal* observed that men of the WIRs 'generally dislike ardent spirits', and Robert Armstrong, head of the naval hospital in Jamaica, agreed with Richardson that while 'rum is cheap in all the islands, an instance of intoxication among the negroes is seldom met with'. To those accustomed to white troops, whom some described as being 'addicted to drinking', the fact that WIR soldiers were 'generally sober' and did 'not drink as the whites' was remarkable.[95] There is some data to confirm this general impression. During the two years the 4WIR were in Gibraltar, just four men were court-martialled for drunkenness, whereas the comparable figure for the 26th regiment was forty-eight men.[96]

Richardson disagreed with those who suggested black soldiers lacked the opportunity to imbibe to excess, or possessed 'an instinctive feeling, that the wants of the system do not require such stimulating substances'.[97] In fact, despite the sobriety of the 4WIR in Gibraltar, plenty of other WIR

[92] See Trevor Burnard, *Mastery, Tyranny and Desire: Thomas Thistlewood and His Slaves in the Anglo-Jamaican World* (Chapel Hill: University of North Carolina Press, 2004).

[93] Report annexed to the annual abstract of sick, Windward and Leeward command from 21 December 1822 to 20 December 1823, WO334/2, 30. The garrison surgeon in Sierra Leone in 1831 reached a similar conclusion. Annual report on prevailing disease in the West African command for 1831, WO334/7.

[94] Report on creation of the WIRs written by R. Blackworth, 10 February 1836, 39 CO320/3. See also Churchill, 'Efficient, efficacious and humane responses', 143.

[95] Inspection reports for 4WIR 1812, 1WIR 1819, 6WIR 1812 in WO27/113 and WO27/147.

[96] Inspection reports for 4WIR and 26th foot, WO27/147.

[97] 'On the utility and economy of the West India regiments', *United Service Journal* (1833), pt 2, 494. Robert Armstrong, *The Influence of Climate and Other Agents on the Human Constitution* (London: Longman, 1843), 22. See also Fergusson, 'On the qualities and employment of black troops in the West Indies', 523.

soldiers were court-martialled for being drunk on duty. Richardson himself reported that 'African and coloured soldiers of the 2 W India Regt have not only the same means of indulging in intemperate habits that soldiers generally have, but are particularly exposed to this vice from having been so many years quartered in a town where they are surrounded by grog shops in which spirits can be had at the lowest rate'. During the seventeen years he had served in the West Indies, Richardson had witnessed many black soldiers 'drink very hard and sufficiently to render some of them fatuous ... yet during thirty years spent principally within the tropics I never witnessed a case of delirium tremens occurring in a black man'.[98]

Since, in his opinion, immunity to 'delirium tremens' extended to the wider black population, Richardson believed there must be 'physical differences in the situation of the black man, and in his mental and bodily constitution that render him less liable to this disease'. As the skin of the black man was widely accepted to be of 'greater density' than that of Europeans, Richardson theorised that 'the membranous and vascular structure of the brain' was likely similarly structured, helping to prevent the 'bodily and mental exhaustion' that were typical of delirium tremens. The immunity from fatigue in tropical climates thus made black men 'constitutionally' resistant to delirium tremens. In addition to a physical defence, Richardson believed that the black soldier also had 'a degree of apathy that renders him almost invulnerable to compunctions leveraging on distressing states of mind and so long as he can get what he requires for daily sustenance he is insensible to despondency and those depressing poisons that effect the drunkard'.[99] Benjamin Moseley agreed that the black soldiers were 'not subject to nervous diseases. They sleep sound in every disease; nor does any mental disturbance ever keep them awake'.[100] This, of course, concorded with racialised tropes about 'happy' black people, lacking the higher brain functions of the white man, whose singing and dancing were proof of their contentment with slavery and other forms of unfree labour.[101] The cheerfulness of Africans, both enslaved and enlisted, was thus given an innate physical cause, one that biology dictated.

---

[98] Reports into Delirium Tremens, 9 March 1841, WO334/174. Twelve members of the 1WIR and eighteen members of the 5WIR were punished for drunkenness in the first six months of 1812. WO27/108.

[99] Reports into delirium tremens, 9 March 1841, WO334/174.

[100] Moseley, *A Treatise on Tropical Diseases*, 492.

[101] See, for example, James Walvin, *Questioning Slavery* (London: Routledge, 1996), 116; David F. Ericson, *The Debate over Slavery: Antislavery and Proslavery Liberalism in Antebellum America* (New York: New York University Press, 2000), 25; James Oakes, '"Whom have I oppressed?" the pursuit of happiness and the happy slave', in James Horn et al. (eds.), *The Revolution of 1800: Democracy, Race and the New Republic* (Charlottesville: University of Virginia Press, 2002), 220–39.

The list enumerating the ways in which the bodies of black soldiers were an improvement on white counterparts kept on growing. They were largely immune to tropical fevers; the after-effects of hard drinking common to all soldiery seemed as nothing; they were brave and committed, especially when originating from one of the particularly martial West African ethnic groups; and their thicker skin seemingly helped to prevent injuries and allowed wounded men to recover rapidly. Commanders who worked with the WIRs in the field quickly added another special quality: the stamina and endurance of African soldiers in tropical conditions was highlighted as one of the most significant advantages they possessed over white troops. Even before the end of the eighteenth century, it had become 'a doctrine, commonly maintained by military men, that European soldiers are not capable of undergoing the fatigues of field service in the tropical climates of the West Indies'.[102] Nothing during the ensuing decades persuaded the army that this situation was about to change any time soon. 'Over-exertion; [and] imprudent exposure to the sun' meant that 'European troops, on first encountering a tropical climate, are soon miserably reduced in physical strength', and this was aside from the impact of any endemic fevers. Within months 'many young and gallant fellows' were condemned to an early grave. Black soldiers, by contrast, could readily 'endure the burthen and trial of the service', particularly 'the duties that must be done in the day, when the heat of the sun is so injurious to Europeans'.[103] As the ability to undertake arduous work in tropical heat was something readily attributed to the enslaved population in the West Indies as well, it is not that surprising that black soldiers were believed to possess the same trait.[104] The wives of WIR soldiers, described by one surgeon as 'certainly as hardy' as their menfolk, were thought to share this ability, and their supporting role as 'carrier, forager, cook and washerwoman' made the difference between 'a cheerful and willing or a discontented force'.[105] Luke Smyth O'Connor, an officer who served with the 1WIR in the Caribbean and later in Africa, singled out the men's 'powerful frames and iron constitutions' which enabled them to march in tropical conditions without flagging.[106] Moreover, it was not just that they could do such work,

---

[102] Robert Jackson, *An Outline of the History and Cure of Fever, Endemic and Contagious* (Edinburgh: Mundell and Son, 1798), 75.

[103] 'On the utility and economy of the West India regiments', 493–4.

[104] See Long, *History of Jamaica*, II, 412, and Seth, *Difference and Disease*, 267.

[105] Fergusson, 'On the qualities and employment of black troops in the West Indies', 525.

[106] O'Connor, 'Suggestions for the discipline, uniform, messing and recruiting of the West India Regiments', 362.

some believed black soldiers positively enjoyed it. Lieutenant Colonel
Nathaniel Blackwell, commanding part of the 1WIR on Marie Galante
in 1808, praised 'the cheerfulness with which they went through the
long and harassing marches'.[107]

Not only were black soldiers seemingly possessed of greater stamina
than white soldiers, field commanders also thought they excelled at
field craft, praising 'their ability to penetrate the inaccessible fastness
of the islands to which rebellious slaves were wont to retreat'.[108] In the
early years of the St Domingue campaign, British officers hoped that
'the black troops will acquire a decided superiority over the opposing
brigands, will pursue them into their woods and fortresses, and finally
subdue them. While the towns and posts will be garrisoned by his majesty's regular forces'.[109] In St Lucia black troops were sent against rebels
'to drive them from their retreat on a mountain; which being judged to
be a service of more fatigue than danger, was a proper enterprize on
which to employ the blacks'.[110] This significantly understated the hazardous nature of tracking maroons in the densely forested mountains,
where traps and ambushes quite possibly awaited the unwary. Tracking
maroons was a highly skilled pursuit and evidently beyond most white
regiments. Jamaicans had used 'trusted' slaves for this purpose for a
while, thinking them remarkable 'for tracking in the woods, discerning
the vestige of the person, or party, of whom they are in quest, but the turn
of a dried leaf, the position of a small twig, and other insignificant marks,
which an European would overlook'.[111] Thomas Hislop, commanding
the 11WIR in Guyana, was adamant that black soldiers 'from their constitutions and natural habits' were ideally suited to the light armament
and rapid movement of light infantry.[112] But in reality hunting maroons
required even lighter armament and faster movement than a regular unit
of light infantry could manage. The reputation of WIR soldiers as skilled
trackers capable of rapid mobile warfare led them to be used to suppress
slave revolts in Barbados in 1816 and Demerara in 1823. The conduct
of 1WIR in Barbados in 1816 earned them, according to one eyewitness,
'the admiration of every body and deservedly'.[113]

---

[107] Report of Lt. Col. Blackwell, WO1/96.
[108] Report on creation of WIR written by R. Blackworth, 10 February 1836, 39
CO320/3.
[109] Williamson to Dundas, 13 September 1794, WO1/60.
[110] Vaughan to Dundas, 31 January 1795, WO1/83. Ten years previously the Carolina
Corps had been tasked with dealing with the Black Caribs of St Vincent. Lincoln to
Sydney, 8 March 1784, CO 260/7.
[111] Long, *History of Jamaica*, II, 408.
[112] 'Hislop's Remarks', 28 WO1/95.
[113] Extract of a private letter, 27 April 1816, CO 28/85.

Luke Smyth-O'Connor fleshed out in more detail why he thought native Africans were naturally suited to this form of highly mobile warfare. Prefacing his comments by stating that complex military manoeuvres would probably 'addle' the brains of the 'wild untutored savages' under his command, he argued this actually played to their strengths: 'Their former mode of life…has already initiated them into the leading features of the light-infantry exercise – quickness of eye and movement, vigilance against surprise, coolness and steadiness in firing, and an accuracy in trailing their enemy that can only be acquired by the children of the vast Zahara. A leaf turned, a twig broken, the pressure of the grass, fifty atoms, that would be overlooked or pass unheeded by a European eye, causes the wary savages to halt and escape the ambuscade'.[114] In essence he thought Africans possessed hyper-attuned senses able to perceive crucial details that would be missed by whites. O'Connor's account seems to be based on his personal observations and not simply a repetition of a racial trope. In his 1799 *Account of the Natural Gradation in Man*, Charles White had cited the work of German researchers claiming that optic nerves 'are uncommonly large in the African', granting them superior vision, but the extent to which this idea percolated popular consciousness is debatable.[115] Only one edition of White's book was published, and while it was an important contribution to the medical and ethnological literature, the claim regarding eyesight was not widely cited by others. It seems unlikely that military officers writing decades later were swayed in their opinion because of it. Excellent eyesight was a very useful trait for any soldier, and therefore it was entirely natural for commanders to comment on it. The keen vision of black soldiers meant that 'as marksmen they were superior to the ordinary run of white soldiers', and while the men of the 3WIR were sometimes observed to 'overshoot their distances', this was attributed to 'a degree of impetuousness, celerity and impatience in the character of the black troops'. Overall, most regimental inspectors thought 'they fire uncommonly close and well'. Major General Edward Couran, inspecting the 2WIR in Jamaica 1817, reported 'their dexterity and quickness in firing, levelling and loading struck me forcibly'.[116] Thus not only were WIR soldiers naturally equipped to cope superbly with tropical service, they seemed to be innately skilled in one of the principal duties of a soldier.

---

[114] 'Suggestions for the Discipline', 362.
[115] White, *An Account of the Natural Gradation in Man*, 80–1; see also Mark M. Smith, *How Race Is Made: Slavery, Segregation and the Senses* (Chapel Hill: University of North Carolina Press, 2006), 12 and Winthrop Jordan, *White over Black: American Attitudes towards the Negro* (Chapel Hill: University of North Carolina Press, 1968), 501.
[116] Report on 3WIR 1812, WO27/108; 2WIR 1817, WO27/141.

Hearing was another sense that was crucial for a soldier, since instructions were often conveyed via the use of bugle calls or drumbeats. Commanders believed that WIR soldiers possessed better hearing than white soldiers, indeed 'the negro's ear is proverbial for its accuracy'. Another aspect of heightened hearing much appreciated by WIR commanders was the regimental bands. The innate musicality of those of African descent was a commonly held trope in the Americas. Even Edward Long, who thought Africans completely 'void of genius', conceded 'they have good ears for music'.[117] Those dealing with the WIRs echoed and amplified this idea. Nearly every inspection report singled out the musicians of the WIRs for praise. Major General William Monro, inspecting the 1WIR in Trinidad in 1812, reported a 'very fine corps of drummers, and also a most excellent band of musick'; at the headquarters of the 6WIR in Martinique the musicians were 'very good, fully competent to their duty'. Excellent musicians led one commander to praise 'the soldier-like appearance and correctness of movements in the field' of the 6WIR.[118] Beyond that, the band was involved in a variety of ceremonial occasions such as funeral processions and marching from port to barracks, and even sometimes gave concerts for the wider population.[119]

Military surgeons serving in the West Indies had therefore made a key contribution to debates about differences between white and black bodies. Michael Joseph has argued that black soldiers were valued 'not for any absolute physical qualities like strength, but rather for their ability to undergo the necessary extremes of fatigue without succumbing to disease'.[120] But the evidence suggests that innate physical qualities were precisely what both commanders and physicians appreciated. Unlike most eighteenth-century Caribbean physicians, army surgeons believed that physical and medical differences between white and black soldiers were actually far more than just skin deep. Skin was important, crucial in fact, but evidence of physical differences was everywhere, even in the eyes and ears of black soldiers. Importantly, the consistent commentary they provided in both private reports and published accounts, depicted the soldiers of the WIRs in a largely positive light. From their mental acuity which, with a bit of time and training, had the potential

---

[117] Long, *History of Jamaica*, II, 353, 423. On hearing, see also Smith, *How Race Is Made*, 12, and White, *Account of the Regular Gradation*, 81.
[118] Report on 1 and 6WIR 1812, WO27/113.
[119] Elizabeth Cooper, 'Playing against empire', *Slavery and Abolition* 39 (2018), 540–57.
[120] Michael Joseph, 'Military officers, tropical medicine, and racial thought in the formation of the West India regiments, 1793–1802', *Journal of the History of Medicine* 72 (2017), 159.

to match European soldiers, to their stamina and physical strength that ideally suited them to mountainous and densely wooded environments, their almost superhuman senses that provided better sight, hearing and hand-eye co-ordination, and their proven martial skill and bravery, black soldiers far exceeded the abilities of white counterparts. Given the continued understanding that black troops were 'fever-proof' in locations where fever was both endemic and unavoidable, it is not surprising that one surgeon who twice served in the Caribbean described the WIR 'as fine a military corps ... as ever was seen of any colour'. He predicted that 'hereafter Great Britain, unless she means the same tale of woe to be rehearsed for ever, must condescend to conquor, and more especially to preserve her conquests, with the black man's instead of the white man's arm'.[121] As we shall see in the next chapter, these ideas about the special abilities of black bodies became so pervasive that they became the most important determinant in how WIR soldiers were treated.

---

[121] Fergusson, *Notes and recollections of a Professional Life*, 208; 'Dr Fergusson on yellow fever', *Medico Chirurgical Review* 32 (1840), 303.

3   The Use and Abuse of the Black Soldier

The observations of regimental surgeons and commanders, as reported to superiors in London and periodically published in medical journals or as stand-alone volumes, shaped a narrative between c. 1795 and c. 1830 that WIR soldiers had unique physical abilities. It was not training that forged the men of the WIRs into ideal soldiers, rather it was biology, or put more simply race. It was their black skin that made them resistant to disease and wounds alike and gave them the stamina to withstand and even enjoy tropical heat. Their better vision and hearing allowed them to excel at soldierly tasks. This racialised, and explicitly medicalised, interpretation of the bodies of WIR soldiers as articulated by physicians rapidly seeped into the consciousness of their commanding officers and increasingly infused every aspect of their treatment.

All soldiers, whether black or white, were expected to reside in barracks provided by the army. Barracks helped to 'introduce among them discipline and regularity' and offset the allure and temptations of taverns and brothels that might be nearby.[1] Not all barrack accommodation were the same, however. Some forts were in isolated locations, and buildings were often not in the best state of repair. Medical personnel stationed in the Caribbean frequently commented on the location of barracks and in particular cautioned against those built in, or close to, swamps. The problem with swamps, as one physician noted, was that they were 'much troubled with insects' and everyone knew that 'places much infested by insects are always unhealthy'.[2] Theodore Gordon, inspector of hospitals in the Windward and Leeward Islands at the start of the nineteenth century, observed: 'The positions of the barracks in several of the colonies, altho' they may be eligible for the purpose of defence, are very objectionable in a medical point of view, and undoubtedly heighten

---

[1] Adjutant General Hope to Governors of Grenada, St Kitts and Dominica, 23 January 1797, WO1/86.
[2] William Fowle, *A Practical Treatise on the Different Fevers of the West Indies* (London: H. D. Symonds, 1800), v.

84

the proportion of mortality'. He believed that high mortality rates were unavoidable 'as long as European troops are quartered on the sea coast and especially in the towns of the West Indies'. The answer, now that the WIRs were up to full strength, was to allocate barracks by race since 'it is a singular fact that the positions healthy to the European prove sickly to the African, and those which are healthy to the African are fatal to the European'. European troops should be posted to mountains in the interior and avoid the coast. 'The African on the contrary is vigorous and healthy on the sea coast, but becomes indolent and liable to frequent and severe diseases in the mountains, the air of which to his constitution is comparatively cold and damp'.[3] Gordon's message evidently resonated in military-political circles in London. 'Antigotham', writing in *Cobbett's Political Register* a couple of years later, agreed that only black regiments could occupy coastal forts as the climate 'is not so obnoxious to them'.[4]

Almost as soon as the WIRs were created, commanders began to think of locations where they could handily replace white troops. Prince Rupert's Head in Dominica, for instance, was perhaps the best strategic location in the West Indies, but also one of the unhealthiest, being adjacent to a large swamp that acted as a breeding ground for mosquitos. Even before the new strain of yellow fever appeared in 1793, British officers on the island knew the 'exceedingly unhealthy' situation meant 'a stationary regiment there, will...never be in any strength'.[5] Thomas Reide, surgeon to the 1st regiment of foot that was stationed in the Caribbean in the early 1790s, ruefully recorded that 'the situation of this place is not a healthy one. ... Every regiment which has been quartered there has been unhealthy, and lost a number of men'.[6] It was at locations such as these where black troops came into their own. Henry Dundas recommended that 'the garrison should be composed, in as great a proportion as possible of black troops, whose health I am assured is seldom affected, or in a very slight degree only, by the causes which render this spot so frequently fatal to Europeans'.[7] Thus at Prince Rupert's, and in many other locations known to be especially unhealthy to Europeans, the WIRs rapidly replaced white troops. In 1798, for instance, General Cornelius Cuyler reported he had sent 'half of O'Meara's corps [later

---

[3] 'General return of the sick and wounded ... from December 1799 to January 1803', CO318/32.
[4] *Cobbett's Political Register*, 23 February 1805, 287.
[5] Meyers to Mathew, 4 September 1791, CO101/31.
[6] Thomas Dickson Reide, *A View of the Diseases of the Army in Great Britain, America, the West-Indies and On Board of King's Ships and Transports* (London: J. Johnson, 1793), 182.
[7] Dundas to Cuyler, 10 January 1798, WO1/86.

part of the 12WIR], a fine body of men from St Lucia to Trinidad, from whence I have ordered a detachment of the 3d infantry which has been much reduced by sickness'.[8]

Throughout the early nineteenth century, the choice of postings for all regiments serving in the West Indies continued to be dictated by medical theories as to which were the healthiest locations for each race. Indeed, one of the main rationales for continuing with the WIRs, after the peace with France and the end of the external threat to British islands in 1815, was that 'they can garrison unhealthy posts for years, where white men would perish in a few months'.[9] In Demerara the fact that white troops were 'dispersed along the East Coast, leaving George Town to be garrisoned by Black troops' was explained by the fact that 'George Town, being on the banks of the Demerara River, is not so well exposed to the fresh sea breezes and trade wind, and is therefore looked upon as being less healthy, than the East Coast'.[10] Frederick Bayley, whose father was stationed in Grenada in the 1820s, noticed that white soldiers were housed on Richmond Heights whereas Hospital Hill, 'on account of its unhealthy position,… is used only as a station for black troops'.[11] The Grenada Gazette, recalling that a detachment of the 76th regiment had lost a third of its compliment in Dominica in just eighteen months, praised a proposal to augment the size of 1WIR in 1836 precisely because it would enable them to garrison 'those stations that have proved most destructive to white troops, such as Berbice, Tobago, St Lucia, and Dominica'.[12] Orange Grove barracks near Port of Spain, Trinidad, proved so sickly for white troops the builders 'might as well have dug graves for them at once'. Yet a few years later, William Fergusson 'found a negro regiment living at these barracks in a state of the greatest health and comfort'.[13] In Jamaica, the 2WIR occupied the barracks at Port Royal that had an unenviable reputation 'for plague and pestilence, and to be ordered there seemed equivalent to a death-warrant'. The only white regiment in Jamaica by the 1840s was stationed at Newcastle in the mountainous

---

[8] Cuyler to Dundas, 3 April 1798, WO1/86. This corps would later become the 12WIR.

[9] 'On the utility and economy of the West India regiments', United Service Journal (1833), pt 2, 494.

[10] Observations to accompany the annual return of sick and wounded form the Windward and Leeward island command for 1830, WO334/5.

[11] Frederick William Naylor Bayley, Four Years' Residence in the West Indies during the Years 1826, 7, 8 and 9 by the Son of a Military Officer (London: William Kidd, 1833), 455–6.

[12] Grenada Gazette, 31 December 1836.

[13] Dr William Fergusson, 'On malaria and yellow fever in the West Indies', United Service Journal (1837), pt 3, 379.

interior, 4,000 feet above sea level and well beyond the reach of tropical fevers.[14] Consigning the WIRs to garrison duty at low-lying coastal forts deemed unhealthy for white people inevitably exposed white officers attached to the WIRs to considerable risk. Their vulnerability, compared with the private soldiers, was noticeable. The 3WIR lost sixteen officers when quartered near Kingston, Jamaica, and the 'Serjeant Major and almost all of the white Serjeants' of the 8WIR perished when stationed in Dominica between September 1801 and April 1802. Sickness was also rampant. The white officers of the 8WIR serving at Pointe-à-Pitre in Guadeloupe in 1812 were afflicted by 'perpetual fever and ague attendant on all white people quartered there'.[15]

Allocating accommodation by race was not simply done because white soldiers died too quickly in forts situated close to swampy regions, and thrived in mountainous, airy locations. Some medical personnel believed that black people actually received health benefits from living in such locations. William Fergusson, after many years of West Indian service, argued that 'warm, moist, low, and leeward situations' were 'congenial in every respect' to the black soldier because 'he there enjoys life and health'.[16] Another doctor thought all black people, enslaved or enlisted, 'benefited by living in a low situation, near to marshes, which quickly prove fatal to whites'.[17] High ground, on the other hand, was understood to be dangerous for black people due to the strong 'currents of wind that sweep the mountain tops'. This helped to perpetuate an idea that real kryptonite for the black soldier was cold weather. Chilly temperatures were something he 'cannot bear', cold winds 'had uncommonly severe effects' and wherever situated the black soldier 'always seeks the protection of a closed hut and the cover of a blanket', regardless of how stiflingly hot it was.[18] One regimental surgeon confirmed that WIR soldiers 'scarcely ever sleep, if they can avoid it, in a current of air, they carefully close up every crevice, that can admit the breeze from without, and make an atmosphere

[14] Luke Smyth O'Connor, 'Leaves from the tropics', *United Service Journal* (1848), pt 2, 334.

[15] William Lempriere, *Practical Observations on the Diseases of the Army in Jamaica as They Occurred between the Years 1792 and 1797* (London: T. N. Longman, 1799), I, 111–13, 165. Major J. Gordon, *Proceedings of the General Court Martial in the Trial of Major J. Gordon, of the Late 8th West India Regiment* (London: E. Lloyd 1804), 61, 155. Report on the 8WIR 1812, WO27/108.

[16] William Fergusson, *Notes and Recollections of a Professional Life* (London: Longman, 1846), 203.

[17] W. M. Harvey and John Lindesay, 'Account of the cachexia Africana: a disease incidental to negro slaves lately imported into the West Indies', *The Medical Repository of Original Essays and Intelligence* 2 (1799), 284.

[18] Fergusson, *Notes and Recollections*, 207. John Williamson, *Medical and Miscellaneous Observations Relative to the West India Islands* (Edinburgh: Alex Smellie, 1817), 117.

agreeable to themselves, that would in many instances produce serious disease in Europeans'.[19] By situating the WIRs as far as possible from what Europeans would consider welcome and refreshing breezes, military authorities were continuing to show faith in the idea that black bodies were uniquely adapted to thrive in warm coastal environments.

WIRs were often allocated badly built and poorly maintained barracks. After all, it had become common parlance that black soldiers had thicker skin than whites and if black skin was sufficient to turn the point of a lancet, as regimental physicians suggested, it would surely provide extra protection against the elements as well. Comfortable accommodation would simply be a waste of resources. When the formation of the regiments was being discussed prior to 1795, one officer argued that there was little need to pay 'great attention to good quarters' for black recruits since 'the worst species of encampment [would be] superior to the protection they are in general afforded in the islands'.[20] That might have been true as a generality, but there are plenty of examples of pitiful shelters for the WIRs. The first detachments sent to Honduras in 1797 were forced to plead for 'pavilions' to protect them from the 'myriads of musquitoes and sandflies'.[21] Matters had only improved marginally by 1808. The 5WIR, still in Honduras, was now housed 'in little detached huts in swamps to which access is only to be had by plank or embankment', and for three months each year there was barely 'a piece of dry ground to stand upon'.[22] The problem facing commanders was that relieving the 5WIR with anything other than a different WIR would highlight 'the disadvantages that any regiment must labour under in that station'.[23]

The 5WIR's hospital in Honduras was situated 'in a swamp, to leeward of extensive morasses, inundated by the sea...in the very metropolis of sand-flies and mosquitoes'.[24] It would be hard to find a worse location for those already sick. Hard, but not impossible. In Guyana the military hospital for both black and white soldiers was leeward of a marsh where 'aquatic larvae and exuviae abounded, and over them clouds of

[19] Army Medical Department: Returns and reports observations on the diseases treated in the Detachment Hospital in Barbados from 24 May to 25 December 1823 by Mr Deed, WO334/2.

[20] Add MS 28062 (fol 378) [1787] British Library.

[21] Cummins and Cavenagh to Barrow, 4 October 1797, WO137/99.

[22] Confidential report on 5WIR Belize, 21 November 1808, WO1/95.

[23] Carmichael to Gordon, 8 January 1809, WO1/95. For other examples of poor accommodation, see the Report of 1WIR 1807 in Barbados, where the barracks were described as 'extremely bad' and one building had been condemned, WO27/90; and the 'dilapidated state of the buildings' occupied by 1WIR in Antigua in 1828, *Antigua Weekly Register*, 28 October 1828.

[24] O'Connor, 'Leaves from the tropics', pt 3, 224.

mosquitoes and sand flies... almost every case admitted to this hospital during the epidemic became yellow fever, no matter what the ailment on admission; and it ultimately became such a terror to the soldiers, that the utmost difficulty was experienced in persuading them to enter it when sick'.[25] Those determining the layouts of military installations rarely consulted regimental surgeons, much to their frustration, and if surgeons proffered advice they were often ignored. When William Fergusson was inspecting facilities in Trinidad and was shown the proposed location of the 'principal barracks', he 'considered it [his] duty to point out its insalubrity'. His advice had the opposite effect from what he intended: 'One would have supposed from the event, that instead of protesting against, I had actually recommended it, for the building of the barracks was commenced forthwith, at an enormous expense, and to the certain destruction of all white troops that have ever been made to inhabit it'.[26]

Newly built barracks were invariably reserved for white troops, with black troops left to occupy second-hand buildings that had often been erected in haste. In 1823 military labourers attached to the 1WIR in Barbados were housed in barracks made 'of wood, seated on low land very near the sea and... in a bad state of repair'.[27] Twenty years later the accommodation for black troops had not improved. The Dockyard Barracks consisted of 'two long, low, narrow wooden buildings, running parallel to the sea and to each other, and about four feet above high-water mark. A pond, originally intended for seasoning spars and timber, ranges between the buildings, which, if not constantly attended to, emits a foul and unwholesome effluvia'. Only black troops occupied such unpleasant barracks, since it was accepted 'they are not calculated for Europeans' who, by contrast, required 'the protection of solid walls in apartments raised off the ground'.[28] In Trinidad 'there are two posts which ought always to be occupied by black soldiers', Governor Hill reported, 'the ordnance store barracks at Cocorite encompassed with a miasmatic swamp, and the sea fort battery flanked to the Windward by the mud swamp of the river'.[29] By 1837 these 'old and fast-decaying'

[25] Daniel Blair, *Some Account of the Last Yellow Fever Epidemic of British Guiana* (London: Longman, Brown, Green and Longmans, 1850), 6.
[26] Fergusson, *Notes and Recollections*, 67–8.
[27] Army Medical Department: 'Returns and reports annual report on the diseases which have occurred at the Head Quarters of the 1st West India Regiment at Saint Ann's Barbados for the period from the 21st December 1822 to the 20th December 1823', 10 WO334/2.
[28] Luke Smyth O'Connor, 'The command in the Windward and Leeward Islands', *United Service Journal* (1843), pt 2, 93; William Fergusson, 'On barrack accommodation in the West Indies', *United Service Journal* (1838), pt 1, 89.
[29] Hill to Glenelg, 10 November 1837, CO295/114.

barracks, built by the Spaniards more than forty years previously, were the home of the 1WIR. As early as 1799 these barracks were deemed to be 'unhealthy', and such poor accommodation undoubtedly had an impact on the health of those living there, with the regimental surgeon commenting that 'the proportion of sick is greater than it would be were the men quartered in better barracks'. Unsurprisingly, the new 'very expensive' barracks built near Port of Spain were reserved for white troops.[30] J. Hall, staff surgeon on St Vincent, was somewhat taken aback 'that the black troops at Old Woman's Point have more than double the space allotted to them than the white troops have in Fort Charlotte'. In his experience white troops always had the superior accommodation, but his request to have some white troops moved to share accommodation with the 1WIR was denied. The government of St Vincent, responsible for the upkeep of Old Woman's Point, had refused to fund repairs, and when the 1WIR arrived it was a 'ruin and the greater part were completely without walls'. The men had therefore decided to undertake repairs 'at their own expence and by their own manual labour'. The commanding officer did not think it was fair to re-appropriate the barracks now they were habitable.[31]

Surgeons perceived a clear link between poor-quality accommodation and disease, and at least some recognised that even their superhuman black soldiers suffered by living there. A detachment of the 2WIR stationed in the Bahamas in 1830 was divided between newly constructed barracks in Nassau and the old barracks at Fort Charlotte, which were 'fast falling into decay'. The old barracks were 'of course becoming annually more unhealthy for the troops', while the men at the new Barracks 'still continue to enjoy, comparatively, a much greater exemption from disease than the others'.[32] With West Indian barracks being of such variable quality, one surgeon went so far as to recommend doing away with them completely. William Fergusson suggested to the commander in chief in the Windward and Leeward Islands in 1817 that WIR soldiers 'should be made to hut themselves'. Since most WIR recruits, he thought, had been accustomed to constructing their own accommodation 'before they came into our hands', they would probably 'be comfortable and happy' in 'a well-ventilated, healthy habitation' of their own construction instead of being housed in barracks.

[30] Trigge to Dundas, 20 March 1799, WO1/87; Report on the 3WIR 1822, WO27/155; Sir Andrew Halliday, *The West Indies: the Natural and Physical History of the Windward and Leeward Colonies* (London: John William Parker, 1837), 318.
[31] Hall to Winchester, 27 December 1841 and reply. Wellcome Library MSS RAMC/397/B/CO/2.
[32] Annual Medical Report of the 2nd W India Regt for 1830, WO334/5.

An added bonus was that it 'would eminently prepare them for the warfare, that of woods and mountains, to which they are destined'.[33] In the West Indies, at least, this suggestion was not taken up.

Differential treatment can also be discerned with regard to diet. The rations issued to WIR soldiers were initially the same as those issued to white troops in the Caribbean, and a typical weekly ration consisted of 5 pounds of bread, 2 pounds of fresh meat, 2 pounds of salt beef, 27 ounces of pork, 9 ounces of sugar, 10 ounces of rice, 5 ounces of cocoa and 2.5 pints of peas.[34] Regimental surgeons persistently tried to alter a diet that they considered to be unsuitable for those of African descent. William Fergusson cautioned that it was a mistake to assume that the newly regimented African 'shall at once have the appetites and digestive organs of his new estate, and exchange his vegetable diet of the fruits of the earth for salt beef and rum'.[35] Theodore Gordon, in overall charge of military hospitals in the Windward and Leeward Islands, recommended in 1803 that the diet of WIR soldiers should instead be 'composed principally of farinaceous and vegetable substances, <u>with only a small portion of salted animal food</u>; a diet much more consentaneous to their constitutions and habits of life, than the present'.[36] A vegetable-based diet was deemed to be naturally suited to African digestive systems, and Robert Armstrong, head of the Naval Hospital in Jamaica, believed that meat-rich European diets were actually physically harmful to black soldiers. He observed that 'among the blacks in the West Indies, the quantity of animal food consumed is much less than the ration of a European soldier; yet, when these men enlist, they are at once placed upon a highly nutritious diet, to which they have never been accustomed, and which the wants of the system do not require: plethora is the consequence, and a greater liability to disease'.[37] Although the rapid change of diet was generally blamed for any increase in the number of recruits reporting sick, few surgeons held out any prospect that black stomachs were actually capable of adapting to a European diet. Armstrong does not make it clear whether he thought black soldiers might, ultimately, become accustomed to this diet, but

---

[33] Fergusson, *Notes and Recollections*, 212.

[34] Alexander M. Tulloch, *Statistical Report on the Sickness, Mortality and Invaliding among the Troops in the West Indies; Prepared from the Records of the Army Medical Department and War-Office Returns* (London: W. Clowes and Sons, 1838), 5.

[35] Fergusson, *Notes and Recollections*, 210. See also Wendy D. Churchill, 'Efficient, efficacious and humane responses to non-European bodies in British military medicine, 1780–1815', *The Journal of Imperial and Commonwealth History* 40 (2012), 141–3.

[36] 'General return of the sick and wounded ... from December 1799 to January 1803', CO318/32.

[37] Robert Armstrong, *The Influence of Climate and Other Agents on the Human Constitution* (London: Longman, 1843), 106.

he seemed adamant that black bodies 'do not require' the same calorie intake as white ones. Just as black skin marked Africans as being externally distinct from Europeans, their internal organs were increasingly accepted to be fundamentally different as well.

Some took the advice from surgeons immediately on board: when Governor Andrew James Cochrane-Johnstone sent black soldiers against maroons in Dominica they were ordered to 'root out and destroy [their] provision grounds, leaving only what may be of service to a detachment of 30 men of the 9th West India Regiment ordered to occupy one of the camps until further orders'.[38] Evidently the food grown by maroons would be perfectly suitable for the 9WIR. In the Bahamas WIR soldiers received far less salted meat than their white counterparts, since 'it has been found that they suffered even more from a salt meat diet than the whites'. Extra rations of rice and peas were substituted.[39] Some commanders instructed the quartermasters of the WIRs to avoid 'giving them false appetites' since they actually preferred 'the simplest and commonest food'. In any case the wives of married men tended to barter away their official rations 'for food...to suit their husbands' palates and habits'. In Grenada, according to one report, 'one day's salt provisions in every week, are sold, or exchanged for vegetables'. Replacing meat with vegetables would also reap health benefits: 'The physical strength of the men would not be diminished by a change of food; on the contrary, if possible, increased'.[40]

In an effort to get the policy adopted, some highlighted the potential cost savings of reducing or eliminating meat from the diet of black troops since 'the produce of the country is their natural food' and they could be expected to grow their own food and forage for extras.[41] This placed the men in a similar situation to the enslaved population, who used garden patches to grow vegetables and established a thriving trade in foodstuffs and other items on most West Indian islands.[42] Increasing

---

[38] Johnstone to Portland, 4 September 1800, CO71/32.

[39] Tulloch, *Statistical Report on the Sickness, Mortality and Invaliding among the Troops in the West Indies*, 72.

[40] Luke Smyth O'Connor, 'Suggestions for the discipline, uniform, messing and recruiting of the West India regiments', *United Service Journal* (1837), pt 1, 363. Report for the 6WIR WO27/90.

[41] Add MS 28062 (fol 378) British Library.

[42] Sidney W. Mintz and Douglas Hall, *The Origins of the Jamaican Internal Marketing System* (New Haven: Yale University Press, 1970). Neville Hall, 'Slaves use of their "free time" in the Danish Virgin Islands in the later eighteenth and early nineteenth century', *Journal of Caribbean History* 13 (1980), 21–43. Woodville K. Marshall, 'Provision ground and plantation labor in four Windward Islands: competition for resources during slavery', *Slavery and Abolition* 21 (1991), 48–67; Hilary McD. Beckles, 'An economic life of their own: slaves as commodity producers and distributors in Barbados', *Slavery and Abolition* 21 (1991), 31–47.

the amount of vegetables and rice in the diet of WIR soldiers would be 'cheaper' than providing either fresh or salted meat, and would prove a 'great saving of the public purse, as well as of their own health'.[43] In the absence of an official policy, however, implementation was patchy. As late as 1840 rations for troops in West Africa were 'the same for the black as for European troops' but with a new emphasis on fresh instead of salted meat. The policy was roundly criticised by doctors, and 'the change experienced by the Negro, from the vegetable or farinaceous diet commonly used among tropical nations, to one principally composed of animal food, and that of a very stimulating description' was blamed for the rapid increase in bowel disease among black troops.[44] The partial implementation of the recommendations of army surgeons suggests that this particular issue was left to the discretion of individual commanders, and for some it was far simpler to issue the same rations to all soldiers.

Not content with attempting to influence what entered black bodies, surgeons also had opinions on their external coverings. When the idea of recruiting black troops was being discussed, some years before the WIRs were actually founded in 1795, one factor deemed to be in their favour was that less clothing would be required and therefore 'some saving might be made'.[45] But when the WIRs were formally constituted, it was accepted that they should 'be in all respects upon the same footing as the marching regiments', and this meant the standard regimental uniform. Numerous paintings from the early nineteenth century depict the WIR soldier wearing a uniform that would clearly have marked him out as a British soldier on the battlefield (Figure 3.1). The coat was the usual bright red, and the tall hat and white trousers could be found among the uniform of several other British regiments. There was little visually to distinguish the WIRs from other regularly established regiments, itself an important visual statement that the WIRs were a fully integrated part of the British army. Not all the clothing was new – when the 4WIR were posted to Surinam in 1806 they were forced to put up with 'old caps of different corps', and when the same regiment arrived in Gibraltar in 1817, they were given second-hand shirts from the departing regiments they replaced. The policy of regularly shifting the WIRs to different islands, and splitting them into small

---

[43] Fergusson, *Notes and Recollections*, 211.

[44] Alexander M. Tulloch, *Statistical Report on the Sickness, Mortality and Invaliding among the Troops in Western Africa, St Helena, the Cape of Good Hope and the Mauritius; Prepared from the Records of the Army Medical Department and War-Office Returns* (London: W. Clowes and Sons, 1840), 17.

[45] Effingham to Grenville, 19 March 1791, CO137/88.

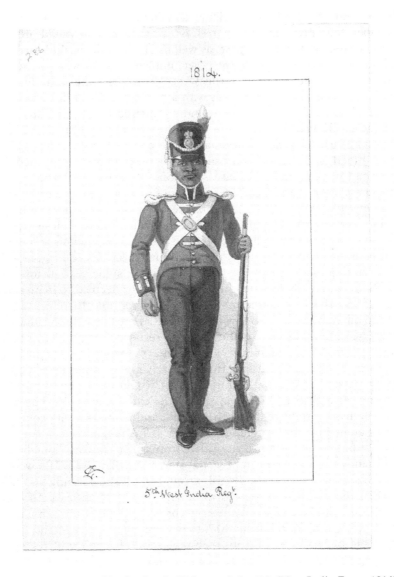

1814.

5ᵗʰ West India Regt.

Figure 3.1 Charles Lyall, 'Private of the 5th West India Regt. 1814'. Prints, Drawings and Watercolours from the Anne S. K. Brown Military Collection. Brown University Library.

detachments, meant new clothing was often late arriving. The commander of the Leeward Islands complained in 1807 that 'the want of clothing' for the WIRs had been mentioned in each of his two previous reports, while the detachment of 4WIR garrisoning St Maarten in 1813 had missed out on new supplies in both 1811 and 1812 and was still wearing the tattered remnant of uniforms from 1810. Matters improved after 1815 when there were fewer WIRs and the war was no longer the most pressing matter the army had to deal with.[46]

William Fergusson thought the policy of supplying standard uniforms was entirely wrong. He argued that WIR soldiers 'cannot bear the irksomeness of heavy clothing during the day' and indeed 'would go naked all the day long, if allowed'.[47] Fergusson did not go so far as to propose dispensing with uniforms entirely, but recommended any light clothing as suitable, noting that the preference for bright colours among WIR soldiers meant 'it cannot be made too gay'.[48] Luke Smyth O'Connor, who served with 1WIR for more than twenty years, agreed that the red uniform was 'not suited for purpose', arguing that a green uniform would offer better camouflage.[49] Army commanders paid little attention to these suggestions. The WIRs would continue to wear the usual uniform of a British regiment until 1858, when they adopted the Zouave uniform that would mark them out as highly distinctive within with the British army for the remainder of their existence (Figure 3.2).

More support came from commanders regarding footwear. The army provided shoes but WIR soldiers did not always wear them, and commanders were not overly worried about the situation. General Thomas Trigge reported in 1800 'that black soldiers in general, do not make use of shoes, nor indeed, would it be proper that they should, for it would deprive them of one great advantage which they possess over the white troops', namely, rapidly traversing difficult terrain in pursuit of any enemy, whether French or rebellious slave.[50] The bare soles of African feet, Edward Long claimed, 'by constant exposure, acquire the colosity and firmness of a hoof' and rough terrain held few terrors for them.[51] For Long, black feet adapted as they constantly traversed rough terrain. By the 1830s the emphasis has shifted somewhat. It was not that black feet adapted, they were now seen as intrinsically

[46] Report of the 1WIR and 4WIR 1806, WO27/90; Report of the 4WIR 1813, WO27/108; Garrison Orders Gibraltar, 20 March 1817, WO284/20.
[47] Fergusson, Notes and Recollections, 207.
[48] William Fergusson, 'On the qualities and employment of black troops in the West Indies', United Service Journal (1835), pt 1, 527.
[49] O'Connor, 'Suggestions for the discipline', 362.
[50] Trigge to Dundas, 20 November 1800, WO1/90.
[51] Edward Long, History of Jamaica (London: T. Lowndes, 1774), II, 380, 412.

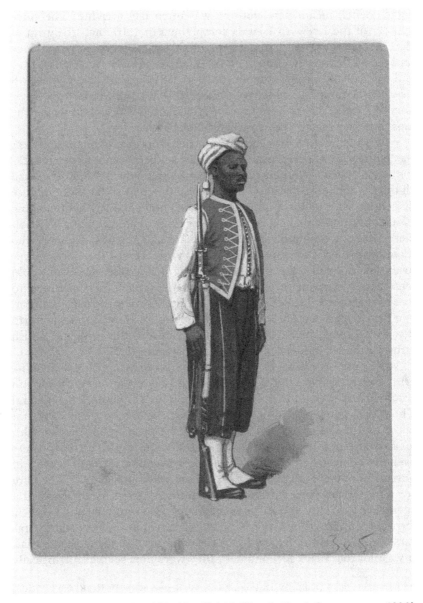

Figure 3.2 Richard Simkin, 'British West Indian infantryman, c. 1890'
(1890). Prints, Drawings and Watercolors from the Anne S. K. Brown
Military Collection, Brown University Library.

unsuited to footwear and shoes not only were unnecessary, they were positively harmful. Knowing that his soldiers 'delight in perfect and unrestrained freedom for their toes', Luke Smyth O'Connor recommended sandals instead of boots.[52] While not going as far as one West Indian physician who insisted that black feet were 'less adapted for walking', William Fergusson accepted that 'the army shoes ordinarily issued to the troops are anything but adapted to the foot of the negro, which is flat, thin, and spread out to a great degree – with toes, that, were they as long, would radiate as wide as the outstretched fingers'.[53] Not only was 'squeezing his flexible, prehensile, flat, horny-soled, spreading foot into heavy English shoes, taken at random from the commissary stores...as preposterous an act of maiming as ever was committed', it was also a simple waste of resources. Fergusson recalled that 'it was a barefooted negro corps that in the insurrection at Barbados, when I was there in the year 1816, first, and easily, overtook the insurgents, and extinguished at once the bellum servile'.[54] Going barefoot was thus promoted as being a viable option since black feet, unlike white feet, were deemed to be incompatible with shoes.

Eschewing footwear left WIR soldiers vulnerable, however. When the governor of Dominica sent out detachments from the 9WIR to attack maroon bands in the interior of the island, his only casualties were 'a few men wounded severely in the feet by the pickets planted in the ground near the camps'.[55] The garrison surgeon in Barbados accounted for an unusually large number of leg ulcers treated in 1823 by pointing out that 'the men, when off duty, particularly the blacks, are in the habit of going without shoes which of course exposes them to accidents in feet and legs'.[56] And assessing the impact of the WIRs in 1836, one report referred not only to 'accidents to their feet' but also 'a complaint in the toes called the "chigoe".'[57] The female chigoe flea burrows into unprotected feet to lay eggs and can cause serious infections. Newly imported Africans, Edward Long reported, were 'seldom free' from an infection of chigoes, and Benjamin Moseley observed that 'the negroes often let them collect and remain in their feet, until their toes

[52] O'Connor, 'Suggestions for the discipline', 362.
[53] James Thomson, *A Treatise on the Diseases of Negroes as They Occur in the Island of Jamaica* (Jamaica: Alex Aikman, 1820), 5. Fergusson, 'On the qualities and employment of black troops', 527–8.
[54] William Fergusson, 'Dr Fergusson's remarks on the statistical report on the sickness &c among the troops in the West Indies', *United Service Journal* (1838), pt 3, 239.
[55] Johnstone to Portland, 4 September 1800, CO 71/32.
[56] Report Annexed to the annual abstract of sick, Windward and Leeward Command from 21 December 1822 to 20 December 1823, WO334/2, 31.
[57] Report on the creation of the WIRs, 38 CO320/3.

rot off'.[58] It was Moseley, it should be recalled, who reported that black people were insensible to pain.

The accommodation, diet and clothing that would have been provided for a white regiment were therefore refined to suit notions of what was suitable for a black regiment.[59] Most of these changes saved the army money, but they were only rarely promoted for economic reasons, and sometimes the army went out of its way to put in special measures for the WIRs that were simply not required for a white regiment. Since most early recruits into the WIRs were purchased directly from slave ships, and the minority who were from the Caribbean had often come from newly conquered French islands, it was hardly surprising that regimental commanders struggled with the fact that most men 'do not understand English'.[60] Soldiers could originate from anywhere along a 3,000-mile stretch of the West African coastline, from Gambia to Angola, with some coming from as far as Madagascar, and probably would not have been able to understand their fellow African-born soldiers let alone European languages. Over time a hybrid language emerged, using elements of European and African languages, though commanding officers continued to complain that it was 'difficult to be understood but by those who are accustomed to hear them speak'.[61] The situation was not entirely hopeless. In each regiment there were a few recruits from English and French Caribbean islands who at least could be expected to understand oral instructions. The muster records of the 7WIR suggest a fairly even split between African and West Indian recruits, with French and Dutch islands predominating. Indeed, the commander of the 8WIR in Guadeloupe in 1812 remarked that it was unusual that his NCOs 'speak less of English or French than any other black corps I have met with, therefore strangers must find it difficult to understand them'.[62]

The language barrier was considerable but surmountable with a little effort, patience and some sign language, at least to the degree necessary to make basic instructions understood. A bigger problem for the army was illiteracy since 'it rarely happens that a black sergeant or corporal can write or read'. The inability to receive and follow written instructions on active service led one commander to remark, 'I should be very shy of trusting

---

[58] Long, *History of Jamaica*, III, 883; Benjamin Moseley, *A Treatise on Tropical Diseases on Military Operations*, 4th ed. (London: T. Cadell, 1804), 28–9.
[59] R. L. Blanco, 'The development of British military medicine, 1793–1814', *Military Affairs* 38 (1974), 7.
[60] 5WIR 1812, WO27/113.
[61] 1WIR 1817, WO27/142.
[62] 8WIR 1812, WO27/113. WO25/2744.

to their intelligence by confiding to them any separate command'.[63] The 'essential' solution advocated in 1811 by the head of the army, the Duke of York, was the establishment of regimental schools. Hoping that the 'greatest advantages may result from the attention to the instruction of young black soldiers', he suggested one of the black sergeants receive extra pay to act as schoolmaster.[64] The impact of the order was not immediate. Several commanders reported in 1812 that they had been unable 'to procure a fit person to take charge' of a school. In occupied French and Dutch territories the civilian population was unable to help. The 7WIR was stationed in Curaçao, and there was 'no one in the regiment capable of the undertaking and neither can any person be found in Curaçao equal to the duty of the superintendence of a regimental school from the want of perfect knowledge of the English language'.[65] But matters improved quickly, and by 1815 the regimental school in Antigua for the 4WIR had 'fifty seven men and boys learning to read and write, many of them come on extremely well and show much aptitude in learning'.[66] The regimental school for the 1WIR in Barbados was established 'upon the system of Doct Bell', a reference to the monitorial system created by Andrew Bell in Madras in 1790, whereby the most able students would assist in the tuition of the less capable.[67] This helped to offset the difficulty many regiments had previously reported in finding and then retaining suitable schoolmasters. A formerly flourishing school attached to the 5WIR in Jamaica closed in 1815, 'the school master dying on service'.[68] The establishment of schools, and the seriousness with which commanding officers resolved to find teachers and ensure the attendance of recruits, while obviously serving the self-interest of both the army and local commanders, also suggests that black soldiers were thought to be intellectually capable of at least basic instruction.

Those in command of the WIRs clearly accepted and understood the men to be physically different in numerous ways from European soldiers. Their resistance to tropical diseases (attributed to their tougher skin) meant they could occupy posts in unhealthy locations and tolerate poorly built and maintained quarters, without suffering the high mortality that would have inevitably occurred in a white regiment. Aside from their

[63] 6WIR 1812, WO27/113.
[64] York to Liverpool, 15 August 1811, WO1/647.
[65] Report of 5WIR and 7WIR, WO27/108.
[66] 4WIR 1815, WO27/133.
[67] 1WIR 1820, WO27/150. It is not clear if Bell's system was ever used to teach Sepoy units in India, though Bell noted that he aimed to support 'the demands of the army and navy' for educated recruits. Andrew Bell, *The Madras School* (London: T. Ensley, 1808), 9.
[68] 5WIR 1815, WO27/1133.

immune systems, however, what commanders valued above all else was the stamina in tropical conditions that black soldiers demonstrated again and again. Officers took pride that their men were 'equal to great exertion' and that they were 'able to do more work in this climate than three times their number' of European troops.[69] Their ability to perform 'fatigues of which the constitutions of European troops are by no means competent in a West India climate' led them to be first recourse when equipment had to be moved, forts needed construction or military roads driven through a densely wooded or mountainous terrain.[70] An added bonus was that 'the labour they are capable of performing' would reduce army expenditure on the hire of enslaved workers.[71] The inability of white regiments to endure 'the labour of marching in that burning atmosphere' was well known in Britain, and several politicians believed the true worth of the WIRs lay in 'the more fatiguing military duties' they undertook, that 'rescued our European troops from duties peculiarly painful and pernicious to them in the torrid zone'.[72] There are some obvious similarities between how WIR soldiers were described and the perceptions of the physical prowess of the enslaved population. James Thomson in Jamaica believed that 'the broadly-expanded chest, the brawny shoulders and well-turned limb, which every day present themselves in the person of the negro, are not the attributes of one destined to pass his days in listless inactivity'.[73] The army valued this sort of heroic physicality just as much as slave owners did.

The famed stamina of black soldiers meant that they were often tasked with undertaking particularly arduous or taxing duties. When most of the white garrison at Fort Charlotte in St Vincent came down with yellow fever, members of the 1WIR were required to shoulder the 'heavy duty' of undertaking all the guard duty for the garrison. The consequence of this was most had only 'two nights in bed' per week, instead of the usual five. Members of 2WIR undertaking guard duty on pestiferous prison ships in Jamaica fared even worse, with just one night in bed per week.[74] Night duty was believed by some to adversely affect 'the health of the white troops',

---

[69] 4WIR 1815, WO27/1133. Nichols to Vaughan, 11 May 1795 WO1/83. See also 'On the utility and economy of the West India regiments', 495.

[70] Dundas to Bowyer, 22 August 1798, WO1/87; Report on the creation of the WIRs, 10 February 1836, 39. CO320-3.

[71] 'Hislop's remarks on the establishment of West India regiments written in the year 1801', WO1/95, 29.

[72] *Cobbett's Political Register*, 23 February 1805; *Parliamentary Debates* 32 (1815), 1254; James Stephen, *Slavery in the British West India Colonies Delineated* (London: Joseph Butterworth, 1824), I, 427.

[73] Thomson, *A Treatise on the Diseases of Negroes*, 7.

[74] Observations and remarks on the quarterly returns of sick of the troops serving on the Island of St Vincent, January–March 1842, Wellcome Library, RAMC/397/B/RR/1; Carmichael to Castlereagh, 10 September 1808, CO137/123.

and it was mooted at one point that men from reduced WIRs should be attached in small groups to white regiments partly to relieve them of night duty.[75] Although not stated explicitly, the expectation that 'two nights in bed are sufficient' for WIR soldiers is reminiscent of Thomas Jefferson's remark that black people 'seem to require less sleep'.[76] As regimental commanders and surgeons became more familiar with capabilities of WIR soldiers, few saw any reasons to revise the widely held opinion that 'the duties for which they are particularly fitted are those of fatigue, whether of marching or labour'. One surgeon even suspected that the black soldier 'is capable of exertions...which we seem as yet to have had but little adequate idea'.[77] Importantly, arduous labour was not understood to be onerous for black soldiers, instead many believed that the men actually enjoyed it. Andrew Johnstone, colonel of the 8WIR, boasted in 1801 that 'since the Regiment was formed, they have been on repeated occasions employed on duties of fatigue which they always performed with spirit and alacrity'.[78] Johnstone's faith in the happy compliance of his men would come back to haunt him less than a year later.

There was an important difference between military labour and ordinary labour, one that WIR soldiers clearly understood. Building or repairing fortifications, or erecting temporary camps, had an obvious military purpose. White soldiers did this type of work all the time. Road building was more opaque. Roads that connected forts were evidently for military use, but roads that crossed mountainous terrain in the middle of islands with only tangential military usage began to seem suspiciously similar to the work that slaves undertook. When Andrew Johnstone took up his post as governor of Dominica in late 1797, he immediately saw the wider potential of black soldiers for this type of work. He had sent a detachment of the Loyal Dominica Rangers, a body that would later form the core of the 8WIR, against a large band of maroons shortly after his arrival on the island. During an eight-week campaign, during which they 'encountered very great hardships and fatigue [and] it almost incessantly rained', the Rangers successfully killed or captured maroon leaders and destroyed their main camp.[79] Fulsome praise from Johnstone for his black troops led the Duke of Portland to direct him

---

[75] *Saint Christopher Advertiser*, 11 June 1822.
[76] 'On the utility and economy of the West India regiments', 495; Thomas Jefferson, *Notes on the State of Virginia* (London: John Stockdale, 1787), 231. See also Luke Smyth O'Connor, 'Twelve months service in western Africa', *United Service Journal* (1845), pt 2, 63.
[77] Fergusson, *Notes and Recollections*, 210, 206.
[78] Johnstone to Portland, 12 May 1801, CO71/33.
[79] Johnstone to Portland, 10 February 1798, CO71/30.

to 'employ detachments of the black troops stationed in Dominica … in opening roads of communication through the uncultivated and mountainous parts of the island'. This act, he believed, would be an 'evident advantage to the colony'.[80] Johnstone relished the chance for his men to prove 'that they will not only fight, but work for their King'.[81]

Portland and Johnstone were civilians and their view of how black soldiers could be used to further the commercial and imperial ambitions for the island differed markedly from military commanders who proved far more circumspect. General Thomas Trigge, the senior officer in the Windward and Leeward Islands, was worried: 'should these people conceive, that it would reduce them to the condition of common slaves, it might, not only be attended with unpleasant consequences, but, totally overturn every thing that has been done with respect to those corps, and be a very likely means to induce them to join the enemy'.[82] Trigge requested clarification from Johnstone as to the precise nature of the work to be done, and how the men were to be accommodated and compensated. Johnstone replied that this type of work was entirely normal for black soldiers, indeed 'the men of the 9th West India Regiment have been repeatedly employed on fatigue duties in all the islands where they have been. … My regiment at Antigua was employed on the public works there'.[83] The men would be paid an extra sum, in addition to their army pay, but it was perhaps Johnstone's casual comment that overnight accommodation would be sought for the men on nearby plantations that alarmed Trigge the most. As well as being used for labour that was often done by enslaved people, black soldiers would even be housed in plantation huts. Trigge ordered an immediate halt to the plans: 'it would be improper, at this time, to take soldiers from the military posts to employ them in making roads'.[84]

What ensued can only be described as a tussle between civilian and military authority. Despite the direct orders of the home secretary, the Duke of Portland, to permit the use of black troops in road building, General Trigge flatly refused to comply until he received confirmation from commander in chief of the army, Frederick, Duke of York. Such an order would free him 'from all responsibility' for such an unwise course of action.[85] At the same time he ordered the 9WIR, 'a regiment

[80] Portland to Johnstone, [25] November 1799, CO71/31.
[81] Johnstone to Portland, 12 May 1801, CO71/33.
[82] Trigge to Johnstone, 17 August 1800, CO71/32.
[83] Johnstone to Trigge, 30 August 1800, CO71/32.
[84] Johnstone to Trigge, 30 August 1800, Trigge to Johnstone, 11 September 1800, CO71/32.
[85] Trigge to Johnstone, 6 May 1801, in Johnstone to Portland, 12 May 1801, CO71/33.

of French negroes', to be replaced in Dominica by the 8WIR, whose colonel in chief was none other than Governor Johnstone. If this experiment was going to happen, then Johnstone would have full ownership of it. The Duke of York ultimately sided with Trigge, and as the king's son his view was decisive.

Unable to use the WIR to build roads, Johnstone turned his attention to the troublesome swamp adjacent to the fort at Prince Rupert's. The peninsula is clearly identifiable in Figure 3.3, jutting out into the sea in the north-west of the island. The swamp constituted almost the entire neck of the isthmus that connected Prince Rupert's to the rest of the island and had long been identified as the source of disease. Henry Dundas had recommended in 1798 that 'the garrison should be composed, in as great a proportion as possible of black troops, whose health I am assured is seldom affected, or in a very slight degree only, by the causes which render this spot so frequently fatal to Europeans'.[86] In actual fact, aware that it was 'by no means proper for white troops', one of Johnstone's first acts on arriving on Dominica in late 1797 had been to garrison it with black troops. The garrison surgeon reported that Prince Rupert's was 'justly considered as one of the most unhealthy spots in the West Indies, and has always proved remarkably so to the British troops stationed there, an endemic fever from marsh exhalations generally prevailing more or less at all seasons, attended with great fatality'. Fortunately, 'the Black troops seem scarcely affected by it' and the health of the black garrison was consistently reported as 'good'.[87]

Ideally Prince Rupert's would have been entirely garrisoned by black troops, but on occasion commanders had to supplement the force with detachments of white troops. In June 1799 the 7WIR was stationed at Prince Rupert's but, as a newly formed regiment 'not much advanced in discipline, it has not been considered proper to entrust the defence of it entirely with this corps' and fifty men from the 45th regiment were added. The impact on the health of the 45th regiment was immediate. They became 'very sickly' and 'suffered exceedingly', and by May 1800 it was decided to replace the 7WIR with the 9WIR, which had 'served with great credit' elsewhere, solely because it would allow the 45th regiment to be withdrawn.[88]

Johnstone first received instructions in April 1800 regarding the 'draining of the morass' which had been 'totally neglected', and in August 1801 the Duke of Portland reminded him of 'the necessity of draining and

---

[86] Dundas to Cuyler, 10 January 1798, WO1/86.
[87] Johnstone to Hobart, 4 April 1802, CO71/34.
[88] Trigge to Dundas, 25 June 1799, WO1/87; Trigge to Dundas, 29 May 1800, WO1/89.

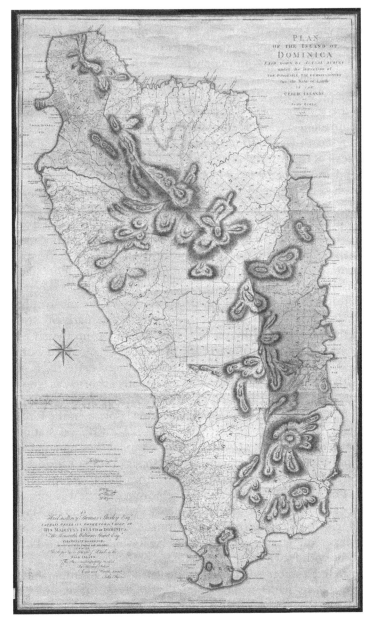

Figure 3.3 John Byres, 'Plan of the Island of Dominica (1776)'. © The British Library Board. Maps K.Top.123.95.a.b.2 TAB. The mountainous interior of Dominica is clearly visible on this contemporary map, as is Prince Rupert's Head in the north-west of the island.

cultivating the swampy grounds adjoining the post of Prince Rupert's and urging him to act 'immediately'.[89] Since the 8WIR were already on-site, General Trigge had 'little doubt' that Johnstone would order the 8WIR to drain the swamp, despite his frequent warnings that 'it would be not only impolitic but hazardous to employ the West India soldiers without paying them in the same manner as the British troops; as any distinction of that sort would be invidious, and could not fail to occasion great discontent, if not desertion; and very possibly mutiny'.[90] In all likelihood Johnstone did not need official encouragement to use black soldiers in these kinds of duties. Aside from an eagerness to prove himself particularly adroit as the colonel of the regiment, and governor of the island, Johnstone also believed that regular labour was good for the men and that idleness was detrimental to their health. When a party of new recruits for the 8WIR arrived in Dominica in 1801, while the main body of the regiment was on active service elsewhere, Johnstone had kept the men busy for three hours a day moving stone for masons building a wall around Government House in Roseau. Crucially, Johnstone claimed he was acting on medical advice as he had been told that it was 'essential for the health of all new negroes, on arriving from a long voyage to exercise men moderately' otherwise the men were 'apt to become sickly'.[91]

From around the middle of March 1802, soldiers from the 8WIR were 'daily employed from the hour of dinner to sunset in cutting down the brushwood in the swamp', equating to about five hours of labour per day, and crucially they did not receive the extra 9d per day that Trigge had ordered should accompany all such work, only an occasional ration of 'extra rum'.[92] Grumbling among the men that they 'were obliged to work like field negroes' appeared immediately and quickly escalated. Governor Johnstone owned land close to Prince Rupert's and the men were well aware that 'the ground of the swamp was the Governor's. Some people said, he was going to build houses on it. Others, that it was to plant canes'.[93] When coupled with rumours, spread by enslaved people from 'adjacent plantations, and at the market, at the town of Portsmouth' that the regiment was about to be reduced as part of a wider shrinking of the army, some made the leap that working in the

[89] Hobart to Johnstone, April 1800, CO71/32; Portland to Johnstone, 20 August 1801, CO71/33.
[90] Trigge to Hobart, 2 April 1802, CO318/19.
[91] Johnstone's Court Martial, WO71/109, 321. For a similar claim, see Long, *History of Jamaica*, II, 433.
[92] Testimony of Sgt Gold Proceedings of Court of Inquiry, CO318/19.
[93] Ibid. Testimony of Corporal Dominique.

swamp was a prelude to enslavement.[94] As one soldier put it: 'now bill hooks were put in their hands, hoes would soon after: that they had carried flintlocks for some time, and would not now use hoes'.[95] These soldiers made a clear distinction between military labour, which might be expected of any soldier regardless of skin colour, and work normally associated with slave labour.

Johnstone had miscalculated what he could order the men to do, and the consequences were severe. On the night of 9 April 1802, just as Trigge had predicted, a mutiny broke out, and within an hour five white officers were dead, others were either imprisoned or in hiding, and the mutineers held one of the most impregnable forts in the West Indies. On hearing the news Johnstone panicked, pleading with Trigge, 'For God's sake send us every assistance you can'.[96] Retaking the fort proved far easier than Johnstone ever dreamed. Gathering the white troops on the island, and with support from the navy, Johnstone travelled as quickly as he could to Prince Rupert's. Messages travelled between the fort and the governor, and professing loyalty to the king, and in the hope of getting a fair hearing for their grievances, the mutineers naively allowed Johnstone and the white troops with him to enter the fort on the afternoon of 12 April. Figure 3.4 depicts the detailed geography of Prince Rupert's Head, with a single access road snaking along the southern coastline to the fort's main buildings. Barracks dot both the inner and outer Cabrits, the two large hills that dominated the peninsula, with the main parade ground located in the valley between them. The 8WIR were drawn up on the parade ground; Johnstone ordered them to lay down their weapons, but some refused and almost immediately a shot rang out. It was not clear who fired first, accounts at the time blamed one of the 8WIR, but a later account by a white officer recalled it was a white soldier who pulled the first trigger.[97] Both sides felt themselves under attack, and what had been a relatively orderly scene descended into chaos. The mutineers fled to hide on the Cabrits, but since 'the red flag was hoisted, indicating that no quarter would be given to those still in mutiny', white soldiers gradually and methodically hunted them down. Any mutineers attempting to reach the sea were shot at by the Royal Navy ships riding at anchor. At dawn the next

---

94 The plan to reduce the number of regiments, including several WIRs, was clearly known in the Caribbean before the mutiny. See the report from Nassau dated 6 March 1802 in the *New York Advertiser* 5 April 1802.

95 Ibid., Testimony of Sgt Gold; Testimony of Capt. Barr and Capt. Cassin.

96 Johnstone to Trigge, 10 April 1802, CO318/19.

97 'The mutiny of the 8th West India regiment from the papers of a veteran officer', *United Service Magazine* (1851), pt 3, 208.

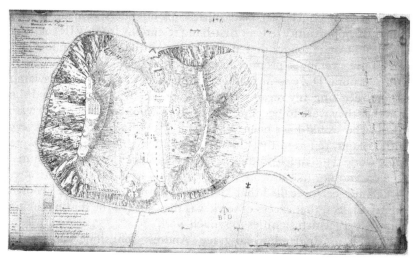

Figure 3.4 'Plan of Prince Rupert's Head 1799', MPHH1/18/1. The National Archives, London.

day, a white flag was raised, indicating surrenders would be accepted, and 'the mutineers began to come in from their hiding places among the rocks and bush'. About a hundred mutineers had been killed, the rest were imprisoned and dispatched by boat to Martinique.[98]

With the fort safely back in white hands, fingers began to be pointed at those thought to be responsible. The legislature of Dominica was of the 'opinion that some glaring misconduct has been exercised towards the 8th West India Regimt', in particular relating to 'pay withheld, and labour unjustly imposed'. The fact that this 'imposition of field labour; in cutting wood for the immediate emolument of their officers' could not have been done without the knowledge and acquiescence of senior officers meant that the colonel of the regiment, Governor Johnstone himself, should be held responsible.[99] The official army enquiry took a similar line, pointing to 'the manner and nature of their employment in working at the swamp' as the root cause.[100] The various investigations,

[98] There are several first-hand accounts of what happened on 12 April. See Johnstone to Hobart, 17 April 1802, CO71-34; *Dominica Journal*, 14 April 1802 (reprinted in *New York Evening Post*, 22 May 1802); Officer from Dominica 15 April (*London Courier and Evening Gazette*, 17 June 1802), 'The mutiny of the 8th West India regiment from the papers of a veteran officer' and 'A further account of the mutiny of the 8th West India regiment', *United Service Magazine* (1851), pt 3, 207–10 and 399–401.

[99] Report of a committee of the Dominica legislature into the state of the colony 17 June 1802, CO71/34.

[100] Proceedings of court of inquiry, CO318/19.

and subsequent courts martial of the leading offenders, provide us with a very rare opportunity to hear first-hand testimony from WIR soldiers. Corporal Strong thought that 'not receiving any compensation for their work at the swamp, as promised them, caused them to be dissatisfied', while Corporal Davy went further, stating that 'working at the swamp without receiving any recompense for their labour' had reinforced the 'idea that they were to become field negroes'. Dominican-born Private Stuart, who would have been well aware of the nature of field slavery on the island, reported that the men had often complained they were 'being worked too much' and, contrary to Governor Johnstone's claims, the men 'did not like to work'. Captain Barr, who was taken prisoner by the mutineers, recalled that 'Sergeant Church told him, in his own country dialect, that excess of work was the cause of the mutiny saying <u>Curry, Curry</u> which signifies too much work'.[101]

Recalled to England in disgrace, Andrew Johnstone was court-martialled by the army in 1805, with one of the charges being that he 'directed the Regiment to be employed in cutting wood, and clearing some swampy ground in the neighbourhood of Prince Rupert's in the island of Dominica, with the view (as would appear) to convert the same to his own use'.[102] The garrison commander at Prince Rupert's, Major John Gordon, initially downplayed the role that working in the swamp had played in the mutiny, informing the court of inquiry at the end of April 1802 that the work had only lasted 'a few days' (several WIR soldiers testified it had actually been ongoing for several weeks) and had amounted to just a couple of hours per day (most WIR soldiers remembered that the work had lasted from around lunchtime to sunset). He claimed to have observed 'no discontent or reluctance' among the men. Three years later, following his own trial and acquittal for causing the mutiny, Gordon's memory had improved and he now accepted that overwork was a 'principal and immediate cause of that unfortunate event' and blamed Johnstone for issuing orders that he did not feel able to ignore.[103] General Trigge testified that he had opposed using black soldiers in this manner several times as first it 'would do away the strong distinction between black soldiers and slaves', and second because it was seen to be 'a considerable duty in the opinion of the soldiers; and I always looked upon the opinion of the black soldiers as of great importance'.[104]

---

[101] All the testimony cited comes from Proceedings of court of inquiry, CO318/19.
[102] Court martial of Andrew Cochrane Johnstone, WO71/109, 3.
[103] Proceedings of court of inquiry, CO318/19; Court martial of Andrew Cochrane Johnstone, WO71/109, 13. Gordon, *Proceedings of the General Court Martial in the Trial of Major J. Gordon.*
[104] Ibid., 199–200.

In his defence Johnstone blamed the munity on 'new negroes' unaccustomed to military life, though regimental pay books confirm that ten of the thirteen men executed for their involvement in the mutiny had been members of the regiment since at least June 1798.[105] He also claimed that the use of black soldiers in these tasks was 'common practice in all the West India Islands' and there was no expectation of extra pay 'when only employed for a short period'.[106] And rather than being resentful of the work, Johnstone disingenuously claimed it 'was considered by the soldiers in the light of a pastime; where for a couple of hours playful occupation in cutting brushwood in the afternoons, they were to have each the allowance of a quantity of rum'.[107] Johnstone's case was entirely in line with his previous claim that the men of his regiment were not only capable but proud to 'work for their King'.

Johnstone was ultimately acquitted by the court martial, mainly on technical grounds, but the Duke of York, the commander in chief, was not so forgiving. He refused to grant the promotion that Johnstone felt entitled to.[108] Perhaps something of Johnstone's character can be gleaned when one looks at his later career. After leaving the army he became an MP for a Cornish rotten borough and devised the Great Stock Exchange Fraud of 1814, deliberately spreading stories of the death of Napoleon knowing the price of government stocks, which he had recently bought, would rise. He made a large profit and fled the subsequent court case, leaving his nephew to face prison and disgrace. He lived abroad for the rest of his life, including spending time in Dominica (where he still had property), Demerara and finally Paris until his death in 1833. Even his own brother described him as a 'an unprincipled villain, swindler and coward'.[109]

For the 8WIR the aftermath of the mutiny was devastating. The regimental return on 1 April 1802 listed 475 privates, 37 black NCOs and 14 white officers. A month later only 374 privates, 28 NCOs and 10 white officers remained.[110] Within two weeks of the mutiny the surviving members had been transported first to Martinique, where the

[105] Court martial of Andrew Cochrane Johnstone, WO71/109, 45; 8WIR Paybooks, WO12/11564 and 11565.
[106] Court martial of Andrew Cochrane Johnstone, 332.
[107] Court martial of Andrew Cochrane Johnstone, 345.
[108] Johnstone published a lengthy exculpatory account complaining about his lost promotion. *Defence of the Honourable Andrew Cochrane Johnstone* (Edinburgh: Manners and Miller, 1806).
[109] David Cordingley, *Cochrane the Dauntless: the Life and Adventures of Admiral Thomas Cochrane, 1775–1860* (London: Bloomsbury, 2007), 237.
[110] Returns for April and May 1802, WO17/2498. Seventy-seven of the privates were listed in May as 'sick', quite possibly wounded in the aftermath of the mutiny.

seven men convicted of active participation in the murder of officers were executed, and then to Barbados where the regiment was solely employed in fatigue duties. Another round of courts martial was held in Barbados resulting in the execution of a further six men.[111] The regiment was disbanded on 24 September 1802, with 148 former members exonerated of involvement in the mutiny being transferred to the 1WIR, 3WIR and 4WIR to continue their lives as soldiers. The remaining 206 men were reduced to the status of pioneers and divided up to serve with white regiments.[112]

The mutiny of the 8WIR almost certainly gave pause to those who considered using black troops in a similar manner. Additional new companies of black pioneers were established and placed at the disposal of white regiments solely for the purpose of 'easing them of the most menial and laborious parts of their duty'. WIR soldiers would never again be asked to undertake the work of slaves, and indeed white officers had to swear an oath that they were not using formally embodied black soldiers for that purpose.[113] The WIRs themselves were too valuable to be done away with, and commanders went out of their way to paint the mutiny as an aberration, triggered by a particular set of circumstances. General Trigge, in the immediate aftermath of the revolt, issued a set of general orders that were distributed to every outpost in the West Indies, stating that 'this unfortunate event will not induce him, in the smallest degree, to suspect the fidelity of the other West India Regiments; he will not confound the innocent with the guilty; and he sincerely hopes that no person will be so unjust as to do so'. He pointedly let it be known that 'detachments from the 4th and 10th West India Regiments... furnish the guard on his quarters: he does not intend to make any alteration, but will continue surrounded and guarded by these troops, with the most entire confidence in their fidelity and good conduct'.[114]

Ideas about black bodies had clearly influenced the treatment of WIR soldiers in a variety of subtle, and not-so-subtle, ways. With hindsight it is evident that the mutiny only occurred because of the prevalent ideas about black soldiers' superhuman resistance to disease and capability for hard work. The 8WIR were only posted to Prince Rupert's Head because it was deemed far too unhealthy for white troops to occupy. They were only sent in to clear the swamp, the unhealthiest part of the entire peninsula, because their colonel in chief thought their robust

---

[111]   Gordon to Johnstone, 30 May 1802, WO71/109, 64v; 8WIR Paybook, WO12/11565.
[112]   Monthly returns for September and October 1802, WO17/2498; Jamaica report c. 1808, CO137/121.
[113]   Jamaica report c. 1808, CO137/121.
[114]   General orders 27 April 1802, CO318/19.

constitutions meant they could undertake such labour in the heat of the day with no physical consequences. At issue was not their capability to undertake this task, it was the propriety of asking them to do it at all.

Assumptions about the nature of the black bodies belonging to WIR soldiers were so pervasive that they gradually seeped into the minds of every regimental commander and surgeon. No matter if the barracks were dilapidated, or adjacent to a foul-smelling marsh teeming with insects, they would suffice for a WIR. Should fresh or salted meat be in short supply, then a WIR would manage perfectly well with just vegetables. If a shipment of clothing had been delayed or gone astray, then the WIRs could make do with cast-offs from others, or in the case of shoes, simply do without. Should a task arise demanding arduous labour in sweltering heat, then the WIRs were always the first to be called upon. It should be stressed that commanders did not do this out of spite: as Chapter 2 established, WIR soldiers were generally held in extremely high regard by their officers. In fact, most of the time commanders treated WIR soldiers differently because they thought the changes were actually beneficial to the men. Instead of looking on a coastal barracks near a swamp with horror, the WIR soldier, it was thought, 'delights in them, for he there enjoys life and health'. If the barracks were completely uninhabitable so much better since the WIR soldier would much prefer to build his own simple hut, reminiscent of his African home, 'where all his affections are centred'. Simple meals consisting of 'the plantain, the yam, the sweet potato, &c', properly seasoned, would result in something 'even the epicure…might envy'. As for working in tropical heat, few would dispute the claim the African soldier 'delights in the sun'.[115] These ideas all coalesced into a broader understanding that Africans serving in the WIRs were 'naturalized to the climate'.[116] It made humanitarian as well as military sense to post the WIR to locations where they were 'vigorous and healthy', and it would be both inefficient and illogical to station them in places that were 'comparatively cold and damp' since the inevitable consequences would be 'frequent and severe diseases'.[117] Many of the medical problems in the WIRs, thought one physician, could be attributed to the 'unnatural mode of living to which we have condemned them' and especially to 'diseases which follow all rash attempts to control nature, and the habits which are justly said to be a second nature'.[118]

---

[115] Fergusson, *Notes and Recollections*, 203–7.
[116] Fergusson, 'On the qualities and employment of black troops', 523.
[117] 'General return of the sick and wounded … from December 1799 to January 1803', CO318/32.
[118] 1817 Report to the commander in chief in the Windward Islands, quoted in Fergusson, 'On the qualities and employment of black troops', 525.

The main intellectual legacy emerging from all the writings of WIR surgeons and commanders in the early nineteenth century was confirmation that the bodies of African soldiers varied from the white norm and merited differential treatment. Old eighteenth-century notions that differences between white and black bodies were minor and largely superficial had been superseded by more than thirty years of empirical observations. WIR surgeons had systematically pointed out the error of treating white and black soldiers alike, and while the army often ignored their advice, the groundwork had been laid for those who came later. Few could claim after reading the works published by John Hunter, Robert Jackson, Benjamin Moseley, William Fergusson and others that black and white men were medically identical. The WIRs were absolutely critical to this intellectual shift. No other men of African descent underwent such medical scrutiny for such a prolonged period, and while much of what army surgeons had to say about the black male body was positive, that nuance was easily overlooked. The key point that became ingrained was that black and white bodies were innately different. The notion that the WIRs were ideally suited to tropical service remained largely uncontested until the end of the 1830s but, as Chapter 4 will explain, the challenge when it came would be immense.

4 Statistics and the Reinterpretation of Black Bodies

The positive narrative about black bodies emerging from those who worked with or commanded the WIRs in the early decades of the nineteenth century began to be reconsidered in the late 1830s. There had always been occasional voices doubting the intelligence, work ethic, fitness and general martial spirit of black soldiers, but these had been generally drowned out by those who wrote, both in public and in private, about their natural suitability for service in the West Indies and their overall military usefulness. Such commentary as there was in the British press about the WIRs tended to emphasise the vital service they were performing in saving European troops from almost certain death. This all changed after 1838, coincidentally the same year as slavery was finally abolished in the British West Indies, as a new narrative emerged emphasising the weaknesses, and in particular the health problems, of black recruits. The articulation of bodily difference so central to the writings of early WIR surgeons was seized on as a conduit for a new, and highly negative, depiction of black male bodies. The two people most directly responsible for this shift were Henry Marshall and Alexander Tulloch.

Henry Marshall was an army surgeon who served in South America, South Africa and finally Ceylon, where he spent thirteen years between 1808 and 1821 serving with the 1st Ceylon Regiment that, like the WIRs, consisted of non-European troops, including a substantial number from southeast Africa. He was appointed deputy inspector of army hospitals in 1830. Alexander Tulloch was a junior officer who joined in the army in 1826 and served in Burma until 1831.[1] Both Marshall and Tulloch shared an interest in the new social science of statistics, which was not the modern-day branch of mathematics, but rather the

---

[1] For biographies, see obituaries in the *Edinburgh Medical and Surgical Journal* 76 (1851), 489–92 [Marshall]; and *United Service Journal* (1864), pt 2, 404–7 [Tulloch]. See also Richard Blanco, 'Henry Marshall (1775–1851) and the health of the British army', *Medical History* 14 (1970), 260–77.

collation and curation of large volumes of data (often by the state). At the formation of the Statistical Society of London in 1834, the Marquis of Lansdowne asserted the goal of the society was 'the collection, not of theories, but of facts, upon which alone all theories and all systems must of necessity be founded'.[2] As one historian has put it, 'Nowhere else was statistics pursued with quite the level of enthusiasm as in Britain' and the curation of medical statistics that would help to 'illustrate the natural history of man in health and disease' became particularly popular. Marshall and Tulloch's work has to be seen as one of the most significant early achievements of this broader movement.[3]

Although limited amounts of data relating to army mortality had been collected and reported since the late eighteenth century, the creation of the Army Medical Board in 1815 vastly increased the volume and quality of the statistics being gathered by the army. Director-General Sir James McGrigor ordered that all regiments at home and overseas submit an annual return listing every medical case treated and its outcome. From 1816 these returns began to arrive at the Army Medical Board, but it took some years before they were subjected to systematic analysis. When Henry Marshall compared the size of force, number of sick and number of military dead in a variety of locations around the world in his 1833 article 'Contribution to statistics of the army with some observations on military medical returns', he relied on the monthly data collected by the War Office, not the medical returns sent to the Army Medical Board.[4] The War Office records (many of which are extant in the National Archives) give the actual numbers, month by month, of how many troops were fit or sick, and how many had died or been recruited, but they do not give information as to illnesses or treatments. Alexander Tulloch also made use of these War Office returns when he sought to ascertain the appropriate rate of military pensions that would allow for the hardships experienced by those posted overseas for long periods.[5]

Having demonstrated both an interest in army medical statistics and an aptitude for using them, Marshall and Tulloch were the obvious choices to undertake an inquiry 'into the extent and causes of the sickness and mortality among the troops in the West Indies, with a view

[2] *Times*, 17 March 1834.
[3] Theodore M. Porter, *The Rise of Statistical Thinking* (Princeton: Princeton University Press, 1986), 24, 37.
[4] Henry Marshall, 'Contribution to statistics of the army with some observations on military medical returns', *The Edinburgh Medical and Surgical Journal* 40 (1833), 36–44, 307–21.
[5] A. M. Tulloch, 'Observations on military pensions, and calculations of their value', *United Service Journal* (1835), pt 2, 145–79.

of founding thereon such measures as might appear likely to diminish the great loss of life annually experienced in these colonies'.[6] Viscount Howick, son of Prime Minister Earl Grey and number two at the War Office, had been tasked by Secretary at War Lord Glenelg with assessing the 'comparative efficiency' of black and white troops in the West Indies. War Office data showed that black troops were less of a financial burden on the Empire than white troops, principally because less needed to be spent on their medical care. Moreover, 'the severity of the colonial service and the consequent rapid wear of the constitution of the British soldier' meant that 19 per cent of British troops had to be replaced every year, whereas only 4.5 per cent of WIR soldiers needed replacing. The medical data Howick had to hand suggested that 'upon an average of ten years the lives of nearly 1/7th of the whole effective force in Jamaica have annually fallen a sacrifice to the baneful effects of the climate, while of the black troops during the same years in the same island the mortality has not quite amounted to 1/27th of the average strength in each year. Even this difference, striking as it is, is very far from showing to its full extent the pernicious influence of this climate on the constitution of the British soldier'. This information only pointed in one direction: 'on the grounds of humanity' the West Indian forces should be 'composed of natives of a tropical climate', by which he meant, of course, those of African descent, rather than the very small number of creole whites born in the Caribbean.[7] Howick was cautious, however. The data he was working from was incomplete, and he recommended to Glenelg that 'further enquiry' should be made into the subject. The appointment of Henry Marshall and Alexander Tulloch was the result.

It took Marshall and Tulloch three years to produce the first of four reports, first on the West Indies (1838), with subsequent volumes appearing on Britain and the Mediterranean (1839), Africa (1840) and Ceylon and Burma (1841). No equivalent volume for India was produced since military forces there came under the control of the East India Company. This was a major research undertaking because, for the first time, the pair had access to the Returns and Reports of the Army Medical Board, an archive that, at the time, consisted of 160 folio volumes. The volumes contained an annual report 'by every medical officer in charge of troops… detailing the number of troops under

[6] Alexander M. Tulloch, *Statistical Report on the Sickness, Mortality and Invaliding among the Troops in the West Indies; Prepared from the Records of the Army Medical Department and War-Office Returns* (London: W. Clowes and Sons, 1838), iii.

[7] Howick to Glenelg, 18 January 1836, WO4/729.

his charge, with the admissions into hospital and deaths among them, in the course of the year, and a specification of the diseases by which they were occasioned'. Medical officers distinguished between officers, rank and file, women and children in the returns, allowing Marshall and Tulloch to see 'whether all classes are affected by the climate in an equal degree', and by including weather data the 'influence of the seasons on the health of troops' could be ascertained.[8]

One vital piece of data was missing from the annual returns of medical officers – the race of the sick and deceased soldiers. Since one of the issues that Marshall and Tulloch had been asked to investigate was any differences 'between the diseases of the white and black troops', they were forced to use a different set of records, the Medical Quarterly Returns, which differentiated between black and white diseases and mortality to create annual equivalent statistics, and then add them to the annual returns.[9] Neither the Medical Quarterly Returns nor the Annual Reports from Stations Overseas seem to survive to the present day, and without Marshall and Tulloch's work, we would have very little direct evidence as to the variations in mortality among troops based in the West Indies and elsewhere.

The first volume, published in 1838, covered the West Indies and, as Marshall had left London in 1836 to be replaced by Assistant Surgeon Thomas Balfour, it was published under Tulloch's name alone. In an overview of the medical statistics for the Windward and Leeward Islands between 1817 and 1836, Tulloch reported that, on average, white soldiers were hospitalised every six months (or twice annually), and 8.5 per cent died each year. In the same years troops stationed in the United Kingdom had a mortality rate of just 2 per cent, but Tulloch also pointed out that between 1803 and 1816 average mortality rates in the Windward and Leeward Islands had been 13.8 per cent, so the period since 1817 actually represented a considerable improvement. As might be expected, given the known susceptibility of European troops to yellow fever and malaria, tropical fevers caused about half the deaths, with dysentery accounting for another quarter.[10]

Turning to the black troops, the raw data seemingly supported the conclusions that so many had drawn from similar data since the 1790s. Between 1817 and 1836 black troops were admitted to hospital fewer than once per year (less than half the rate of white troops) and mortality averaged 4 per cent (again, less than half that of white troops).

[8] Tulloch, *Statistical Report on … the West Indies*, iv.
[9] Ibid.
[10] Ibid., 5–7.

This was not the view Tulloch presented in his report. Instead of reaffirming the superior disease resistance of black troops compared to their white counterparts, and emphasising like so many had before him that black soldiers seemed naturally suited to service in the West Indies, Tulloch questioned why the figures were not even lower. Since he had no data on mortality rates among native peoples in Africa, he used population data from around the world to posit that normal mortality rates among indigenous peoples between twenty and forty years of age did not exceed 1.5 per cent. Native troops in Malta, South Africa and India all had mortality rates lower than 1.5 per cent. If the West Indian climate was 'as congenial to the health of the negro troops as that of their native country', then their mortality rates should be nearer 1.5 per cent not 4 per cent and, in a significant leap, Tulloch claimed that this higher rate 'may fairly be attributed to the insalubrious influence of that climate on their constitutions'.[11]

Tulloch thus agreed with those who argued for a more nuanced interpretation of the relationship between climate and disease. Climate remained one of the greatest factors influencing health, but instead of simply drawing a distinction between cold, temperate and hot climates, and highlighting the health risks for people who transitioned between those environments, Tulloch instead used the Army Medical Board's statistics to confirm that finer gradations between the various regions of the globe were necessary.[12] To him, the higher mortality of black troops in the West Indies, compared to native troops in India for instance, was because 'they are for the most part natives of the interior for Africa' and the climate there 'is probably very different' from that of the West Indies. Both might seem torrid to Europeans used to cooler climes, but there were subtle variations in the amount or regularity of rainfall and seasonality. Africans were also accustomed to a continental climate rather than an island one. Tulloch therefore concluded that the 'indigenous races of tropical as well as temperate climates are peculiarly fitted by nature for inhabiting and peopling the respective portions of the globe wherein they or their forefathers were born, the effects of a transition to any other is in general productive of a great increase in the scale of mortality'.[13]

Further evidence that 'the constitution of the negro can be but little fitted to adapt itself to foreign climates' was found by looking at data relating

---

[11] Ibid., 11.
[12] See Suman Seth, *Difference and Disease: Medicine, Race and the Eighteenth-Century British Empire* (Cambridge: Cambridge University Press, 2018), 15; and Katherine Johnson, 'The constitution of empire: place and bodily health in the eighteenth-century Atlantic', *Atlantic Studies* 10 (2013), 444–52.
[13] Tulloch, *Statistical Report on … the West Indies*, 11.

to civilian black populations in the West Indies. In 1837 Tulloch had published an article, 'On the statistics of the negro slave population in the
West Indies', that tried to account for the long-term decline of the black
West Indian population. Population returns from Britain's Caribbean
colonies showed that the death rate exceeded the birth rate by about
3 per cent and that this was largely due to a high mortality rate rather
than a low birth rate. If the situation did not change, the black population
of the Caribbean would be extinct, he claimed, within a century. Digging
deeper into the causes of high mortality, Tulloch noted that while tropical
fevers did not 'produce the same wide-spreading devastation as among
Europeans', it was 'an erroneous idea to suppose that the negro race
are exempt from the fatal influence of fever in the West Indies'.[14] Innate
immunity to some forms of malaria and acquired immunity to yellow
fever did not mean that those of African descent never came down with a
fever. The impact of fever had to be understood in a comparative perspective. Black people fell sick and died less frequently than white people, and
therefore they seemed comparatively healthy by comparison to the 'devastation' visited upon whites. By far the most important causes of excess
mortality, however, among the enslaved and newly emancipated were lung
diseases, including tuberculosis and pneumonia.

Against a background of 1.5 per cent mortality for indigenous populations, the enslaved mortality rate of 3 per cent does not seem particularly different, but to Tulloch it was twice as high as expected and was
proof that 'the negro race perish rapidly in the West Indies, precisely
from the same cause as Europeans do – the climate is unsuited to their
constitution, being different to that in which they or their forefathers
were born'.[15] It was not individual nativity that counted, since a majority of the enslaved population would have been born in the Caribbean
by the 1830s, it was race. Tulloch believed that an individual's suitability for a climate was permanently fixed and determined by ethnic
background. Moreover, 'as the mortality of the negro slave population
is calculated upon male persons of all ages, including old men and
infants, sickly and healthy; whereas that of the troops is calculated upon
persons in the prime of life only', data indicating higher mortality for
the WIRs suggested that black soldiers were 'subject to some deterio-
rating influence from which the slave population are exempt'. Tulloch
was turning the idea that black soldiers were physically robust and naturally suited to any tropical climate on its head. He also threw down a

---

[14] A. M. Tulloch, 'On the statistics of the negro slave population in the West Indies',
British Annals of Medicine 15 (1837), 453.
[15] Ibid., 454.

challenge to abolitionists in Britain. If the 'alleged ill-treatment' of the black population of the West Indies, then newly emancipated, was so bad, how come mortality was actually higher among black soldiers who 'are well fed, well clothed, and every care is taken of their comfort', with duties that 'are by no means of a harassing nature, and the regulations of the service prevent the possibility of ill-treatment'? The only possible explanation, he argued, was that 'there is a decided inaptitude in his constitution to assimilate itself to the climate of other countries than that indigenous to his race'.[16] Philip Curtin has described this as the 'relocation cost' paid by anyone moving from one specific disease environment to another, but the mediocre diet, poor quality accommodation, excessive fatigue duty and physical violence regularly meted out to WIR soldiers so comprehensively documented in previous chapters, surely also played a part.[17] In reality, as Richard Sheridan has pointed out, Tulloch almost certainly undercounted the mortality of enslaved people since there is ample evidence to suggest it was similar, if not higher, than that experienced by the WIRs.[18] But knowing that Tulloch erred does not undermine his importance in the 1830s, since his publications were accepted at face value and repeatedly cited by others as correct and accurate summations of available statistical evidence.

Tulloch agreed with the idea, promulgated by Edward Long, of a microclimate peculiar to each island in the West Indies.[19] Noticeable variations in the mortality statistics for both whites and blacks on each island highlighted 'how marked a difference there is in the effect produced by their climates on the constitution'. White deaths from fever were three times higher in Tobago than the average for the West Indies as a whole, while intestinal illness were seven times deadlier in Dominica than in Antigua. Similar variations were observed in the statistics for black troops. Mortality from lung disease was much higher in St Kitts than elsewhere, more than double that of Grenada for instance; intestinal illnesses were four times more likely to occur in St Vincent and Barbados than in Antigua. The only explanation he proffered was that 'the climate of each colony' must be sufficiently different to be responsible.[20] The geography of Britain's West Indian islands varied considerably, from mountainous (Trinidad, Tobago, Grenada,

---

[16] Ibid., 453–4.

[17] Philip D. Curtin, 'African health at home and abroad', *Social Science History* 10 (1986), 372.

[18] Richard B. Sheridan, *Doctors and Slaves: a Medical and Demographic History of Slavery in the British West Indies, 1680–1834* (Cambridge: Cambridge University Press, 1985), 15.

[19] See Johnson, 'The constitution of empire', 451.

[20] Tulloch, *Statistical Report on the ... West Indies*, 40.

St Vincent, St Lucia, Dominica, St Kitts, Jamaica) to flat, marshy and wet (Guyana, Belize) or dry and sandy (Barbados, Antigua, Bahamas). Even within each island different hyper-microclimates could be found with swampy parts on mainly mountainous islands for example, and it was well known that the sheltered leeward sides of the islands had very different weather to the exposed windward sides.

Reinforcing his previous conclusions about the civilian black population of the West Indies, Tulloch concurred with leading medical and military authorities that fever 'the great source of inefficiency and mortality among the white troops' had 'comparatively little influence upon the blacks'. But this did not mean that fever was an irrelevance. The important word in Tulloch's statement is 'comparatively'. In fact, it was listed as the cause of about a fifth of hospital admissions among WIR soldiers and 11.5 per cent of the deaths. It was only when placed side by side with the data for white troops that the limited impact of fever among WIR troops became clear. Unsurprisingly, given that dysentery was easily spread in unsanitary living conditions, intestinal diseases among WIR troops caused 11 per cent of hospital admissions and 18 per cent of deaths. Tulloch's major medical finding, however, and again reinforcing his earlier work on the West Indian enslaved population, was proof of the greater susceptibility of black troops to lung-related illnesses, particularly tuberculosis. Lung disease accounted for 6 per cent of white and 12 per cent of black admissions to military hospitals, and the difference was even more marked regarding the severity and ultimate fatality of those cases. About 10 per cent of white troops hospitalised for lung complaints died, but for black troops it was nearly 17 per cent. Such was the mortality that lung diseases accounted for 41 per cent of black deaths, easily the greatest single cause. The peculiarly high rate of mortality from lung disease among black soldiers that 'extends to every climate in which they have been employed' led Tulloch to theorise, and remember Tulloch was not medically trained, 'there must be in the constitution of the negro some peculiarity which predisposes him to affections of the lungs'.[21] Modern medical views might point to the insalubrious and overcrowded accommodation afforded WIR troops, as discussed in Chapter 3, as a cause for this excessive mortality, but instead Tulloch ascribed it to a racial susceptibility.

Tulloch was not the first writer to highlight a supposed predisposition of those of African descent to lung complaints. Lunsford Vandell wrote in 1831 about the 'great scourge' of what he termed 'negro consumption' among black populations in the Americas, attributing it to 'inaptitude

---

[21] Ibid., 13.

of climate'.[22] Samuel Morton observed in 1834 that the 'predisposition to phthisis' among black populations in the United States was 'familiar to every American physician'.[23] It is perhaps unlikely that Tulloch read either of these publications; Vandell's article was published in the Kentucky *Transylvania Journal of Medicine and Associate Sciences*, and Morton's book was only published in Philadelphia. Tulloch did not need these medical publications because he had the reports of army surgeons on his desk that were telling him exactly the same thing, providing qualitative support to his quantitative data. Extant medical reports of army surgeons are frustratingly few and far between for the first half of the nineteenth century. Tulloch had access to twenty years of annual reports from surgeons posted overseas, but only a scattered few now survive in the National Archives. They nevertheless give us a taste of the qualitative evidence that Tulloch had absorbed. Edward Tegart, inspector of hospitals in Barbados, wrote in his 1824 report that the WIR under his care were clearly 'ill able to withstand the effects of cold or wet' and that their 'lungs are very susceptible of disease'. Two-thirds of his pneumonia cases were black soldiers. The impact of phthisis was even worse, with two of every three admissions of black soldiers terminating fatally, six times the rate of white troops. This, Tegart hazarded, 'probably arises from the weak and relaxed state of the callilus structure of the lungs not being sufficiently powerful to form and preserve adhesive defences against tubercles which prevent them from spreading'.[24] Tulloch was therefore reading reports from physicians dealing with black bodies on a regular basis, telling him quite clearly that black lungs were different from white lungs, that they were 'weak', and that it was thus both unsurprising and inevitable that they succumbed to lung illnesses. John Richardson, surgeon of the 2WIR in the Bahamas in 1830, described four fatal cases of phthisis in his annual report, three of whom were African-born WIR soldiers. Richardson's assistant, William Holford Watts, serving with a detachment of the 2WIR in Honduras, was unsurprised when phthisis 'so fatal to the black troops' claimed two of the four cases he treated during the same year.[25]

These internal army documents had minimal impact until Tulloch used them, but there were some contemporary British publications

---

[22] Lunsford P. Vandell, 'Remarks on struma Africana, or the disease usually called negro poison or negro consumption', *Transylvania Journal of Medicine and Associate Sciences* 4 (1831), 94.

[23] Samuel Morton, *Illustrations of Pulmonary Consumption* (Philadelphia: Key and Biddle, 1834), 41.

[24] Report annexed to the annual abstract of sick, Windward and Leeward command from 21 December 1822 to 20 December 1823, WO334/2, 19, 22.

[25] Annual medical report of the 2nd W India Regt for 1830; Annual report of the diseases of the troops serving at Honduras 20 December 1830, WO334/5.

reinforcing the idea that black people were peculiarly susceptible to lung diseases. Henry Marshall, Tulloch's early collaborator on this volume, had observed in 1821 that the East Africans serving in Ceylon were 'very liable to pectoral complaints. … Consumption is a very frequent cause of death among them'.[26] James M'Cabe's *Military Medical Reports*, published in 1825, singled out 'pneumonia, phthisis, pulmonalis' as particularly common among black people. M'Cabe was an army medical officer who had served in Trinidad between 1812 and 1817.[27] Similarly, James Clark's *Treatise on Tubercular Phthisis* of 1834 could easily have come to Tulloch's attention. As physician to Queen Victoria, Clark was prominent in London medical circles and had actually worked with the army's medical records, predating the efforts of Marshall and Tulloch. Clark pointed out that the records proved 'the greater prevalence of phthisis and other diseases of the lungs among the blacks than among Europeans in the West Indies'.[28] *The Cyclopaedia of Practical Medicine*, published in 1835, used military medical records for 1822–9 to show that phthisis and other pulmonary complaints accounted for nearly half of the deaths of black troops in the West Indies, compared to only one-eighth of the deaths of white troops.[29] All these writers agreed that nativity was not a relevant factor: black people from East Africa, West Africa and the West Indies were all peculiarly susceptible to lung diseases. To some extent, therefore, Tulloch's work simply added refinement and greater clarity and detail to the conclusions of others, but what made his research far more important, as we shall see, was the widespread dissemination and discussion of his conclusions.

The available data for Jamaica, an entirely separate military command, did not lend itself quite so neatly to Tulloch's purposes. For one thing there had only been a single small detachment of WIR troops stationed on the island for the majority of the period. Less data was reported to the War Office and the Army Medical Board as a result. Several hundred black pioneers, or military labourers, were attached to the various white regiments, but since they were 'less under medical superintendence than regular corps', they were rarely admitted to a hospital until their illness assumed 'a serious, or perhaps fatal aspect'. Based on the limited and somewhat flawed data he did have, Tulloch

[26] Henry Marshall, *Notes on the Medical Topography of the Interior of Ceylon* (London: Burgess and Hill, 1821), 79.
[27] James M'Cabe, *Military Medical Reports: Containing Pathological and Practical Observations Illustrating the Diseases of Warm Climates* (Cheltenham: G. A. Williams, 1825), 43.
[28] James Clark, *A treatise on Tubercular Phthisis* (London: Marchant, 1834), 50.
[29] John Forbes, Alexander Tweedie and John Conolly (eds.), *The Cyclopaedia of Practical Medicine* (London: Sherwood, Gilbert and Piper, 1835), IV, 315.

calculated that average mortality among black troops, both pioneers and members of the WIRs in the Jamaican command was 3 per cent annually. This was better than the 4 per cent calculated for the Windward and Leeward Islands, but his conclusion that 'the climate must be much more favourable to their health' seems somewhat overstated.[30]

Since the Bahamas had consistently proved unhealthy for white troops, the islands were almost entirely garrisoned by troops from the 2WIR. The 7th Fusiliers had arrived in 1802 with 300 men but departed just a year later with only 50, the rest having succumbed to yellow fever. Tulloch attributed this to the 'unhealthy locality of the barracks', since the mortality among white inhabitants of Nassau was considerably lower than that of white troops stationed at Fort Charlotte, ignoring the fact that locals would have acquired immunity to a disease that had been continuously present since 1793. The fort's hospital quickly garnered a reputation for being 'equivalent to a death sentence'.[31] Even the black troops, usually 'little affected' by fevers, 'suffered severely' in these barracks, particularly the lower floors where 20 per cent died. Overall mortality among black troops averaged 4 per cent, notably higher than the 1.5 per cent among the enslaved population in the Bahamas, again reinforcing Tulloch's argument that native Africans did not fare well in the West Indies, even in a location where 'the climate … is, in general, very favourable to the negro race'.[32] British Honduras (Belize), like the Bahamas, was garrisoned by a small number of white troops and a detachment of the 2WIR. Among whites the mortality was lower than average, and the same would have been true of the 2WIR but for the first outbreak of Asiatic cholera in the West Indies in 1836 that claimed the lives of twenty black soldiers. Tulloch attributed the selective impact of cholera on the 'irregular, drunken, and dissipated' lives of the 'negroes and natives' who were worst affected.[33] A little of Tulloch's own disdain for non-whites appears in that statement.

Tulloch's detailed survey of military mortality in first the Windward and Leeward Islands, then Jamaica, the Bahamas and British Honduras, had strengthened a number of established medical tropes. His finding that fever accounted for a large percentage of the mortality of white troops would have surprised few who had paid the West Indies any attention whatsoever in the previous century. Yet some of his other conclusions proved to be far more innovative. The theory of acclimatisation had dominated thinking about voyages and settlement in the

[30] Tulloch, *Statistical Report on the … West Indies*, 50.
[31] Ibid., 73.
[32] Ibid., 74.
[33] Ibid., 78.

West Indies for hundreds of years. Every new arrival supposedly had to undergo a period of seasoning as their body adjusted to the new environment.[34] This seasoning would invariably involve illness, probably a fever, but the reward for surviving the ordeal was increased immunity to further infections from tropical diseases. Black people, as many had noted, also underwent a milder form of seasoning. Army physicians had increasingly questioned the ability of the seasoning process to create a body of consistently healthy white troops, and this had been one of the most powerful arguments in favour of the WIRs in the 1790s. But it was Tulloch's analysis of the statistics from the Army Medical Board that firmly established this point in the intellectual mainstream. By examining the successive reports of regiments that had spent up to a decade in the Caribbean, he declared that 'for nine instances in which the mortality during the first year has been above average, there are twelve in which it has been below it; ... mortality has increased with length of residence in at least as many instances as it has diminished, and that .... the last years appear even more fatal than the first'. Faced with data from Jamaica that seemed to undermine his case, Tulloch blamed epidemics of yellow fever that skewed the figures. Using data for years without widespread yellow fever actually revealed the fourth year of residency as the most dangerous for a white regiment, mainly due to rotation to one of the unhealthier postings on the island. A case in point was the year 1831, when 'no corps or recruits' arrived in Jamaica yet there were 2,462 hospital admissions due to fever. The total number of white troops was only 2,842.

The conclusion that 'troops are likely to gain but little immunity from either disease or mortality by a prolonged residence in the West Indies' was not a theory, or based on personal observations, but simple statistics: 'the figures establish the facts' and the figures did not lie. Aware that he was tearing down an established 'fact' of West Indian service, Tulloch supposed that the idea of acclimation had arisen due to newly arrived corps comparing their mortality rate in Britain (1.5 per cent) with the previous average for the Caribbean (13 per cent), which immediately produced 'a stronger impression of the deadly nature of the climate'. Corps in their second or third year who dipped below the average mortality 'congratulate themselves on having enjoyed what they deem a healthy season'. Tulloch himself was not surprised at what the data revealed. To him it made perfect sense that mortality was

[34] See Mark Harrison, *Medicine in an Age of Commerce and Empire: Britain and Its Tropical Colonies, 1660–1830* (Oxford: Oxford University Press, 2010), 64; Seth, *Difference and Disease*, 94.

higher among soldiers 'who have suffered for a series of years under the most insidious and fatal diseases to which the human frame is subject' than among those with 'the full health and vigour of an unimpaired European constitution'.[35] There is a further hint, in that sentence, that Tulloch thought the 'unimpaired European constitution' was the summit of medical fitness.

Tulloch was fully aware that his study challenged some long-held medical theories related to climate and race. This did not particularly bother him since he was working from hard data, and therefore 'many of the opinions hitherto entertained ... must have been adopted on very inadequate evidence'.[36] The medical returns simply did not support the notion that tropical diseases were caused by high temperatures since some islands were affected to a greater or lesser degree, despite having nearly identical temperature records. Moreover, some years were far deadlier than others even though temperatures were similar, and occasionally the most virulent outbreaks of disease had actually started in the cooler months, not the hottest ones. The idea that an 'excess of moisture' caused disease was also readily dismissed. Jamaica had considerably less rainfall than Guyana yet proved far deadlier to soldiers. Tulloch also noticed that some stations believed the dry season to be less healthy than the wet season. There was some correlation, he admitted, with higher mortality occurring when both high temperatures and high moisture were present.

Those seeking a geographic explanation of high mortality in the West Indies were also disappointed. Proximity to the 'vast forests' of South America had no bearing, since several colonies close to South America, including Guyana which was actually on the continent, proved healthier than islands many hundreds of miles northward. Those who suggested that soil might be a factor were asked to explain how a location could go from being unhealthy to healthy, or vice versa, when the soil remained the same. Tulloch even challenged one of the oldest tropes of medical knowledge in the West Indies, that marshes caused disease, by pointing out that 'the sickness and mortality in British Guiana and Honduras, where swamps and marshes most abound, are considerably less than at Up-Park Camp, and several of the other stations in Jamaica'.[37]

[35] Tulloch, *Statistical Report on the ... West Indies*, 93–7.
[36] Ibid., 101.
[37] Ibid., 102. On marshes causing disease, see Robert Jackson, *A Treatise on the Fevers of Jamaica, with Some Observations on the Intermitting Fever of America* (London: J. Murray, 1791), 49–51; John Hunter, *Observations on the Diseases of the Army in Jamaica* (London: G. Nicol, 1788), 15–17; William Lempriere, *Practical Observations on the Diseases of the Army in Jamaica as They Occurred between the Years 1792 and 1797* (London: T. N. Longman, 1799), 7.

Reluctant to 'venture any theory of our own, which might on subsequent examination prove as futile as those which preceded it', Tulloch limited himself solely to recommending that forts and barracks be located as high as possible, ideally over 2,500 feet, to counter the impact of tropical illnesses. On islands where this was impossible, then the healthiest locations seemed to be 'low sandy tongues of land, or peninsulas jutting into the sea'. Over a number of years these locations had proved themselves preferable to others. After musing whether windward locations were preferable to leeward ones, Tulloch decided the data was inconclusive. The recommendation pertained to white troops, of course, as only they would garner the benefit of being stationed at higher elevations since 'yellow fever is never known beyond the height of 2500 feet'.[38] Tulloch had no suggestions whatsoever to reduce mortality among the WIRs.

As perhaps the largest and most detailed analysis of official army medical statistics to date, Tulloch's work attracted immediate and widespread attention. Although it was compiled as a report for Parliament, it was published as a book complete with numerous statistical tables. Members of the public could purchase it, and copies were placed in libraries in Oxford, Cambridge, London and Edinburgh. For those unable, or unwilling, to purchase the entire volume there were several other opportunities to learn about Tulloch's work. The London *Times*, read by the most influential individuals, reviewed the volume shortly after publication and believed it would have a 'beneficial influence' in reducing military mortality.[39] Tulloch himself addressed the Statistical Society of London on 18 June 1838, when he summarised his work and read large sections of the report verbatim. The *Journal of the Statistical Society*, founded the following year, reprinted the address over the three issues, ensuring dissemination to those members unable to attend.[40] The editor of the *Journal* believed that 'the value of these statistical investigations to medical science are almost too obvious to require any comment'. The most important achievement, however, was not statistical, or even medical, rather Tulloch had opened 'a new passage in the natural history of man'. When medical officers across the Empire supplied comparable data for 'Maltese, Negroes, Hottentots, Cingalese, Malays, and Hindoos', scientists would be able to see 'at one view the diseases to which each of these races are most subject, and the effect of these diseases, as

[38] Tulloch, *Statistical Report on the ... West Indies*, 103.
[39] *Times*, 29 August 1838.
[40] *Journal of the Statistical Society* 1 (1839), 121–41, 216–330, 428–43.

compared with their influence on the constitution of Europeans serving in the same climate'.[41] As far as the editor of the *Journal of the Statistical Society* was concerned, Tulloch had put racialised medicine on a sounder foundation.

The *United Service Journal*, a publication for serving and retired military personnel from both the army and the navy, also quickly took notice of the publication. Tulloch had written for the *USJ* at least twice before, and the editor somewhat proprietorially called him 'our able correspondent' when first mentioning the publication of the book in August 1838.[42] Reviewing the book over two issues, first dealing with white troops, then with black troops, the *USJ* summarised the main conclusions and included lengthy verbatim quotations. Like the *Journal of the Statistical Society*, the editor of the *USJ* thought the major achievement of the volume was that it opened 'an entirely new page in the natural history of man'. Many already knew that the 'sweeping devastation' of yellow fever largely bypassed the black population of the West Indies, but few could have known, he supposed, 'that diseases of the lungs are the great source of mortality among the negro race in the West Indies'. Crucially, Tulloch's book had exposed as a fallacy the notion 'that because the temperature of the West Indies is probably as high as that of his native land the negro is likely to be healthy there'.[43]

Naturally, the greatest attention to Tulloch's work was paid by medical journals and by individual physicians. Some challenged the entire premise of statistics determining medical policy. The patient, some argued, should be treated primarily as an individual, taking into account 'complex, variable, and often hidden' circumstances.[44] Most, however, considered Tulloch's work a real boon for medical professionals. The *Medico Chirurgical Review* was critical of the fact that Tulloch, 'a mere soldier', took centre stage while placing Marshall and Balfour, his two medically trained collaborators, 'completely in the back-ground' rather than being treated as equal partners. Despite this affront to the medical profession, the *MCR* accepted that this 'highly interesting and valuable document' was 'above all praise' and would 'tend to disabuse the mind of many erroneous and some injurious impressions [and] ... assist the progress of medical science'. Summarising the major

---

[41] Ibid., 444.

[42] Tulloch, 'Observations on military pensions, and calculations of their value', 145–79; Alexander M. Tulloch, 'On the mortality among officers of the British Army', *United Service Journal* (1835), pt 2, 145–72. Tulloch did not sign either of these pieces, but they are referred to later as being his work. The *Naval and Military Gazette* was another military publication to review the volume on 21 July 1838.

[43] *United Service Journal* (1839), pt 1, 373.

[44] Porter, *The Rise of Statistical Thinking*, 157–8.

conclusions, the *MCR* made a point of highlighting data that showed black mortality was higher in the West Indies than in Africa 'and consequently, that the West India climate is unfavourable even to blacks'.[45] The *British and Foreign Medical Review*, aware that others might take issue with Tulloch's statistical rather than medical background, conceded that he was better in ruling out causes of mortality than offering new theories. Nevertheless, 'the perspicuity, copiousness, and accuracy of the details, [and] the prudence of the deductions from them, is not surpassed by anything in the records of our art' and showed 'that medical men have much to reconsider in their existing opinions'.[46] The *Lancet* agreed that it was one of the 'most valuable gifts … made to medicine'.[47] Curiously, no one seems to have criticised Tulloch for conducting what was essentially a desktop study. He never voyaged to the West Indies personally, nor met any WIR soldiers, relying solely on the detailed reports submitted to the Army Medical Board.

One of the most widely read medical journals, the *Edinburgh Medical and Surgical Journal*, devoted forty-five pages to a lengthy summary and analysis of the volume. Henry Marshall had been a frequent contributor to this journal, and the editor ensured that his contribution to this 'useful and important' book was acknowledged. The *EMSJ* perceived the main aim of the volume to be slightly at variance with one stated in the book's preface. Instead of simply uncovering the causes of mortality of troops, this research allowed readers to see 'whether the sickliness and mortality of the different races of mankind were not regulated by general laws'.[48] Despite Tulloch emphasising the higher than expected mortality among black troops, the clear conclusion the *EMSJ* drew from this work was that 'it would be desirable to employ in our West India possessions, to as great an extent as may be compatible with the security of the islands and the safety of the white population, black forces'.[49] The *EMSJ* believed the data confirmed that black troops must have some in-built biological advantage because although they 'suffer as well as the white, yet they do so in a degree so much less'. In a region where alcohol-related illnesses were common among whites, the 'natural' temperance of black troops led the journal to question: 'Can any one after this speak of the superior moral and intellectual qualifications of the European or the Caucasian race over the Negro?'[50] Tulloch's work was leading some to rethink their entire understanding of race.

[45] *Medico Chirurgical Review* 30 (1839), 49, 53; 31 (1839), 24.
[46] *British and Foreign Medical Review* 8 (1839), 211–12, 214, 225.
[47] *Lancet* 2 (1838), 575.
[48] *Edinburgh Medical and Surgical Journal* 50 (1838), 425.
[49] Ibid., 466.
[50] Ibid., 466, 433.

The reviews published in the medical journals take on added importance due to their international reach. Some copies of Tulloch's printed volume were sent overseas. Joseph Skey, inspector general of hospitals, sent a copy to the Surgeon General's Office in Washington DC, for example, but there is no evidence that large numbers of the printed text were sold abroad.[51] Reviews, which printed large sections of the book verbatim, were, by contrast, often picked up and reprinted overseas, particularly in the United States. The review from the *British and Foreign Medical Review* was reprinted in the *Boston Medical and Surgical Journal*; that from the *Edinburgh Medical and Surgical Journal* was reproduced in *The Medical Examiner*, printed in Philadelphia. One journal, the *Medico Chirurgical Review*, was printed in New York as well as in London, and had once boasted 'there is not an island in the great West Indian archipelago which this review does not visit'.[52] Tulloch's research, and particularly his summations on differential racial susceptibility to disease, had thus crossed the Atlantic and medical journals were the vehicles that transported it. It did not take long before American authors began to make use of Tulloch's data. When Thomas Lawson published his own comparative report on mortality in the US army in 1840, he naturally cited Tulloch for comparison.[53]

Two physicians, with precisely the West Indian experience that Tulloch lacked, offered their thoughts on his work. William Fergusson, who had spent two sojourns in the Caribbean in the 1790s and the 1810s and had written extensively on the appropriate treatment of both black and white soldiers, thought the report was 'valuable and excellent' and recommended every officer serving in the West Indies should be provided with a copy. Ignorance could no longer be an excuse for housing troops 'in localities long proved to be pestiferous'. The assault on the theory of acclimation, however, went too far he thought. His own personal experience, together with 'melancholy records of every West Indian expedition that has ever left the British shores', was sufficient proof, he thought, to establish that the 'seasoning principle' existed and functioned 'as a safeguard against tropical diseases'. His own experiences confirmed Tulloch's data that 'the blacks are exceedingly prone to pulmonic complaints when exposed

---

[51] *Army and Navy Chronicle*, 26 September 1839, 198. The only US library with a copy seems to be Harvard.
[52] *Medico Chirurgical Review* 3 (1823), 101.
[53] Thomas Lawson, *Statistical Report on the Sickness and Mortality in the Army of the United States* (Washington: Jacob Gideon, 1840), 325, 337.

to cold in elevated localities, or even to the lesser cold of the winter season between the tropics'.[54]

Sir Andrew Halliday's critique was not only far longer than Fergusson's, it was also published separately as a pamphlet. As the deputy inspector general of army hospitals, Halliday's voice was authoritative. He had spent several years stationed in Barbados and British Guiana in the 1820s and late 1830s, and therefore had relevant personal experience. Like others he disapproved of the choice of a 'military subaltern' undertaking a task better suited to a medical officer. The impact on the morale of the army's medical department would not be positive he thought. Furthermore, Tulloch may have produced a volume replete with 'interesting and invaluable' information, but a trained physician 'might have brought into view many causes of sickness and mortality, that can never be discovered by any accumulation of figures'.[55] Having said that, Halliday spent most of his riposte nit-picking over Tulloch's detailed figures, rather than the broader conclusions he came to. Based on his own personal records, he noted, time and again, that his figures for sickness and mortality did not concord with those of Tulloch, indeed 'in no one year do these returns agree', and thus 'what faith can we put in the calculations made from such uncertain data?'[56] While, like Fergusson, he took issue with Tulloch's dismissal of the theory of acclimation, Halliday also accepted that 'it was the locality, and not the climate generally, that principally affected the health of the troops'.[57] Unlike many others who reviewed Tulloch's book, Halliday made no mention whatsoever about Tulloch's conclusions on the vulnerability of black troops to certain illnesses.

With the volume on the West Indies gaining widespread praise and attention, both at home and abroad, Tulloch followed up with three more volumes along similar lines covering the United Kingdom and British territories in the Mediterranean and North America (1839); Western Africa, St Helena, the Cape of Good Hope and Mauritius (1840); and Ceylon, the Tenasserim Provinces and the Burmese Empire (1841). Where he was able, Tulloch continued to emphasise conclusions about disease susceptibility based on race that had peppered his volume on the West Indies. In Gibraltar, for instance, the posting of the 4WIR to the garrison for two years between 1817 and

[54] William Fergusson, 'Dr Fergusson's remarks on the statistical report on the sickness &c among the troops in the West Indies', *United Service Journal* (1838), pt 3, 235–6, 238.

[55] Sir Andrew Halliday, *A Letter to the Right Honourable, the Secretary at War, on Sickness and Mortality in the West Indies: Being a Review of Captain Tulloch's Statistical Report* (London: John Parker, 1839), 2–3.

[56] Ibid., 30.

[57] Ibid., 46.

1819 provided an ideal testing ground for comparative mortality. It had been hoped that the 4WIR 'would prove extremely useful in relieving the British soldiers from such duties as subjected them to exposure during the heat of the day'. Since Gibraltar was considered to have a hot climate, 'it was not anticipated that this transition would materially affect their health'.[58]

Although not mentioned by Tulloch, part of the rationale for posting the 4WIR to Gibraltar might actually have been the periodic incidence of yellow fever. An epidemic in 1804 had killed 894 soldiers of the Gibraltar garrison, and a further outbreak in 1813 killed 397.[59] Due to the usual rotation of military officers among British territories, numerous individuals served in both the West Indies and in Gibraltar. General Thomas Trigge, who had been commander in chief in the Windward and Leeward Islands in 1802 during the mutiny of the 8WIR, was lieutenant governor of Gibraltar in 1804 when yellow fever struck; General Colin Campbell, acting governor during the 1813 outbreak, had previously participated in the invasions of Martinique, Guadeloupe and St Lucia during the 1790s, campaigns involving several of the WIRs. General George Don, governor of Gibraltar throughout the period the 4WIR was stationed there, had previously been colonel of the 9WIR. These men would have been cognisant of the capabilities of the WIRs, and their well-known resistance to tropical diseases.

When the thousand men of the 4WIR arrived in March 1817, they constituted about a quarter of the garrison. By the time the regiment embarked for disbandment in Sierra Leone two years later, 119 men had died, mainly from lung complaints. This equated to a mortality rate of about 6 per cent per year. Tulloch did not think this level of mortality particularly unusual. Indeed 'it very little exceeded the ratio to which the Negro is occasionally subject'. In fact, mortality rates were almost identical to those for other WIRs in the Windward and Leeward Islands in 1819. The remarkable thing was that 'the mortality was at least four times as high as that of the European troops in Gibraltar in the same period'. For Tulloch this was simply 'another striking instance how unfitted is the constitution of the Negro for any other climate than that of which he is the native'.[60] Had Gibraltar experienced an outbreak

---

[58] Alexander M. Tulloch, *Statistical Reports on the Sickness, Mortality and Invaliding among the Troops in the United Kingdom, the Mediterranean and British America* (London: HM Stationery Office, 1839), 16a–17a.

[59] Sir James Fellowes, *Reports of the Pestilential Disorder of Andalusia* (London: Longman, 1815), 450; 'Account of the 1813 yellow fever epidemic', *Edinburgh Medical and Surgical Journal* (1814), 317.

[60] Tulloch, *Statistical Reports on the ... United Kingdom*, 17a.

of yellow fever during 1817–19, then the picture would, of course, have been very different, but without one, white troops appeared to be far healthier than their black counterparts.

Perhaps because Gibraltar was such an important overseas station, yet also one of the nearest to Britain, the experience of the 4WIR had attracted the attention of medical professionals long before Tulloch published his study. Reviewing one publication on pulmonary consumption in 1819, the *Quarterly Journal of Foreign Medicine and Surgery* diverted from the volume in question to comment on the noted vulnerability of those from tropical climes who ventured into cold climates. Using the experiences of 'An English Regiment of West Indian Blacks' in Gibraltar to illustrate the problem, the journal reported that the men immediately complained of the cold and were provided with additional clothing 'to an extent that would have been burthensome to others'. Nevertheless, 'phthisis became prevalent: and we saw many a poor fellow falling victim to that disease, though treated with all the care, and kindness, and hospitality, for which the Rock is now so deservedly remarkable'.[61] John Hennen, whose *Sketches of the Medical Topography of the Mediterranean* was perhaps the most comprehensive study of disease in Gibraltar, declared that pulmonary complaints were so common that they deserved to be termed the 'true epidemic' of the Rock, ahead of fever. He also pointed to the experience of the 4WIR as a good example of 'the effects of climate in aggravating them'.[62]

Arthur Saunders Thomson pre-empted some of Tulloch's conclusions in his University of Edinburgh dissertation examining the link between climate and mortality, which was published as a book in 1837. Without access to the army medical records used by Tulloch, Thomson arrived at remarkably similar conclusions, including using information on the 4WIR in Gibraltar to argue that 'it does not follow … that the negro will flourish in climates having a similar temperature'.[63] This episode was, he claimed, 'the only instance which has come under my knowledge, where a body of natives were transported from the tropical to the temperate regions'.[64] The importance of the WIRs for Thomson was that they allowed him to observe the impact of a specific variable on a large sample, thus eliminating individual susceptibility as a factor.

---

[61] *Quarterly Journal of Foreign Medicine and Surgery* 1 (1819), 269.
[62] John Hennen, *Sketches of the Medical Topography of the Mediterranean* (London: Thomas and George Underwood, 1830), 121.
[63] Arthur Saunders Thomson, *On the Influence of Climate on the Health and Mortality of the Inhabitants of the Different Regions of the Globe* (Edinburgh: John Carfrae and Sons, 1837), 23.
[64] Ibid., 76.

Where Tulloch had the edge over Thomson was the quality and quantity of his data. Even Thomson acknowledged that the materials available to him were 'so limited and imperfect that no very specific result can be deduced'.[65] So while he could make general observations and link them to the known vulnerability of black troops in the West Indies to pulmonary complaints, he lacked the hard data to really prove his case. Tulloch had all the data he needed, and it was his publication in 1838 that was widely reviewed in British and American medical journals. Thomson went on to serve as an army surgeon in India between 1838 and 1847, and his later writings reinforced Tulloch's claim that it was a 'delusive hope' that Europeans might become truly acclimated to a tropical climate. Data from the West Indies, plus his personal observations in India confirmed, he thought, 'the tropical parts of the world are not suited by nature for the settlement of the natives of the temperate zone'.[66]

Tulloch's third volume of statistics covered territories in and near Africa, including British Atlantic and Indian Ocean islands as well as mainland colonies in western and southern Africa. Unlike the first two volumes, Tulloch was forced to work with incomplete and patchy data, mainly due to the high mortality rate among army physicians posted to Africa. The key person responsible for collating and reporting the statistics sometimes perished before completing the task, and thus 'their death has frequently prevented information from being obtained'.[67] What data existed clearly confirmed that West Africa was a highly dangerous environment for white troops. In Sierra Leone, Gold Coast and Gambia, such white troops that were stationed there were hospitalised, on average, once every four months, and nearly half died, mainly from fever. With 'the impossibility of maintaining white troops in such a climate being thus demonstrated, the garrison has, since the end of 1829, consisted entirely of blacks, with the exception of a few European serjeants'.[68] The contrasting immunity of black soldiers to African fevers was plain for all to see.

---

[65] Ibid.

[66] A. S. Thomson, 'On the doctrine of acclimatization', *Madras Quarterly Medical Journal* 2 (1840), 69; Thomson, 'Could the natives of a temperate climate colonise and increase in a tropical country and vice versa?' *Transactions of the Medical and Physical Society of Bombay* 6 (1843), 132. See also David N. Livingstone, 'Human acclimatization: perspectives on a contested field of inquiry in science, medicine, and geography', *History of Science* 25 (1987), 359–94.

[67] Alexander M. Tulloch, *Statistical Report on the Sickness, Mortality and Invaliding among the Troops in Western Africa, St Helena, the Cape of Good Hope and the Mauritius; Prepared from the Records of the Army Medical Department and War-Office Returns* (London: W. Clowes and Sons, 1840), 3.

[68] Ibid., 6.

Philip Curtin incorrectly interpreted Tulloch to be arguing 'that continuous residence in Africa, and not race per se, was the factor most closely correlated with immunity to fevers'.[69] In fact, Tulloch is quite explicit that 'fatal as the fevers of this colony have proved to the white troops, the blacks have been but little affected by them'.[70] The men of the WIRs had not had 'continuous residence in Africa' by any means. Some had been born in the Caribbean, and this was the first time they had been to Africa. Even among the African born, who still formed the majority of WIR soldiers in the 1820s and 1830s, most had served in the West Indies for a time before returning to Africa.[71] Yet the comparative resistance to African fevers was something that Tulloch believed applied to all WIR soldiers. During the 'dreadful mortality' of white troops in Gambia in 1825, 'a detachment of from 40 to 50 black soldiers from the 2nd West India Regiment only lost one man, and seldom had any in hospital'.[72] While accepting their obvious resistance to tropical fevers, Tulloch continued to push his argument that their vulnerability to other illnesses, particularly lung complaints, meant that black soldiers were far from being the superhuman specimens that previous authors had described. Despite receiving rations and accommodation comparable to that of white troops 'and with an income sufficiently ample to procure all the necessaries and even luxuries of life', hopes that 'the negro soldier would be exempt from any greater degree of mortality than other troops when serving in their native country' were dashed. Average mortality for black troops was 3 per cent, double that of British troops in the United Kingdom or Indian troops in India. Thus 'on his own native coast, even with all the advantages enjoyed by the British soldier, the Negro exhibits a liability to mortality for which it is extremely difficult to account'.[73]

Tulloch recognised that the nature of recruitment of WIR soldiers might have affected his figures. Although every care was taken to 'guard against the introduction of sickly or unfit persons into the service', the fact that many new recruits were 'recently liberated slaves', who had probably experienced privation, meant that they perhaps harboured 'latent diseases' not immediately apparent to regimental surgeons who passed them as fit for service. On the other hand, the comparatively

---

[69] Philip D. Curtin, *The Image of Africa: British Ideas and Action* (Madison: University of Wisconsin Press, 1964), 361.

[70] Tulloch, *Statistical Report on ... Western Africa*, 16.

[71] See, for instance, the Succession book of the 2WIR WO25/645 that lists nativity as well as length of service for soldiers.

[72] Tulloch, *Statistical Report on ... Western Africa*, 13.

[73] Ibid., 15.

high mortality among disbanded WIR soldiers in Sierra Leone, where 1,222 settlers dwindled to just 949 between 1819 and 1826, led Tulloch to return to his favoured theory relating to adaptability. Higher mortality was only to be expected when WIR recruits were 'captured negroes originally brought from a distance in the interior, whose constitutions may not be so well adapted for the moist climate of the sea coast'.[74] The story was the same elsewhere in Africa. In Mauritius, imported black pioneers from Madagascar or Mozambique had similar mortality rates to WIR soldiers in the West Indies, due to 'being transplanted to a climate differing so materially from that in which they or their forefathers were born'. In South Africa, the low mortality of Hottentot troops confirmed the theory of hyper-local adaptation. Tulloch naturally attributed their mortality rate of just 1 per cent to them serving in their own country. Only in St Helena was Tulloch's theory brought into serious question. The civilian black population was actually increasing 'a feature which has never been observed in any other British colony', leading him to conclude, rather simplistically, that the island 'must be healthier than Britain'.[75]

Tulloch's final volume, published in 1841, considered the available data for Ceylon and Burma. The returns from neither province provided data of a similar quantity or depth to what Tulloch had worked with previously for the West Indies or the United Kingdom, and therefore the conclusions he could draw were limited. Fortunately, Henry Marshall had himself served in Ceylon and his mortality data, collected between 1816 and 1820, provided at least some basis to work from. The British had taken the island from the Dutch in 1802 and inherited a body of 'negro troops' that had been imported from Goa and Mozambique. These men were embodied in the 3rd Ceylon Regiment (1803–17) and 4th Ceylon Regiment (1810–15) and were apparently 'of stout and apparently healthy frame, from 5 feet 6in to 5 feet 8in high, very muscular, and capable of undergoing great bodily fatigue. Owing to some constitutional peculiarity, they also have the advantage of enjoying comparative immunity from those aggravated forms of fever which were so destructive to the troops in the interior'. Once again, Tulloch attributes higher resistance to tropical fevers to non-white skin, not to a specific African nativity. Yet, as with black troops elsewhere in the Empire, the average mortality rate of 5 per cent among the Ceylon Regiments was 'considerably higher' than for native troops serving in their own country. Even more remarkably, of around 9,000 men

---

[74] Ibid., 15–16, 21.
[75] Ibid., 5a, 16c.

imported by the Dutch for these regiments, 'none of their descendants can now be traced', and of a further 5,000 imported by the British after 1815, 'not more than from 200 to 300 remain; though every care was taken by the importation of negro females to perpetuate their numbers'. For Tulloch it was clear evidence 'that the climate of Ceylon, like that of the West Indies, must be very unfavourable to the constitution of the negro race'. Just as in the Caribbean, it was lung complaints that proved 'exceedingly fatal' for black troops, and this reinforced Tulloch's earlier argument that time and again the data provided by black troops proved the 'extreme inaptitude of their constitution for withstanding transitions of climate'.[76]

Surveying the mass of data presented in his four volumes, Tulloch concluded that only in their native countries were black troops able to enjoy a mortality rate similar to British troops in the United Kingdom. In practical terms this only meant the small number of soldiers stationed at Cape Coast Castle and the Hottentot troops in South Africa. In West Africa, so well suited was the black soldier to that particular environment that even consumption, so deadly elsewhere, was comparatively 'rare'.[77] As the black soldier moved further and further from his homeland, 'the mortality increases till, in some colonies, it attains to such a height as seemingly to preclude the possibility of his race ever forming a healthy or increasing population'. No single local cause could explain this persistent phenomenon: latitude, diet, housing, temperature, rainfall and elevation, could all be variable, but the mortality of black troops remained stubbornly high. In Tulloch's view the evidence of the medical returns rendered it 'impossible...to say where this class of troops can be employed with advantage'.[78] This conclusion contradicted virtually every other individual who had written about, served with or treated WIR soldiers over the previous forty years.

Military surgeons based in the Caribbean believed that Tulloch's data necessitated a re-consideration of old ideas about race and acclimation. Robert Armstrong, head of the naval hospital in Jamaica, was puzzled by the higher death rates Tulloch reported for black troops in the West Indies compared to the newly freed civilian population. As he knew that as a significant proportion of WIR soldiers were Caribbean born by the 1840s, 'they cannot be supposed to possess any peculiarity

[76] Alexander M. Tulloch, *Statistical Report on the Sickness, Mortality and Invaliding among Her Majesty's Troops Serving in Ceylon, the Tenasserim Provinces and the Burmese Empire; Prepared from the Records of the Army Medical Department and War-Office Returns* (London: W. Clowes and Sons, 1841), 43.

[77] Tulloch, *Statistical Report on ... Western Africa*, 17.

[78] Ibid., 18c.

of constitution, which renders them obnoxious to the climate', and therefore 'some cause must exist besides climate alone'. Armstrong eventually blamed a 'highly nutritious diet, to which they have never been accustomed'.[79] Significant alterations to diet, accommodation and postings of white troops in the Caribbean followed Tulloch's publication. Fresh meat was provided more regularly, new military posts were built in healthier locations, the most notable being Newcastle in Jamaica at an elevation of 4,000 feet, and a new system of rotating white regiments back to Europe every three years was introduced.[80]

Tulloch's career went from strength to strength on the back of these publications. In the 1850s he was chosen to investigate the high mortality experienced by the army during the Crimean campaign and eventually attained the rank of major general, but he only revisited the wider topic of military mortality once more. Using data for 1844–5, Tulloch was pleased to observe a notable decline in mortality for white troops in the West Indies. In Jamaica mortality was actually lower among white troops (2.9 per cent) than among the WIR stationed near Kingston (3.1 per cent), something he attributed to 'important changes ... made in the localities where the white troops were stationed, and in the frequency of reliefs which now take place'.[81] These changes had been made as a direct result of the recommendations in his first report in 1838. The mortality for black troops had, perhaps unsurprisingly since there had been no material changes in their situation, remained virtually unchanged. These 'negroes captured in slave ships, or inhabitants of the West coast of Africa' were, he wrote, simply unsuited to the West Indian climate and 'their constitutions never have, and probably never will, become assimilated to it'.[82]

In his publications Tulloch had challenged the entire basis for the use of black troops within the British army. From the 1790s through to the 1830s, the majority of those writing about WIR soldiers had considered them to be a major benefit to the Empire, able to serve in locations that had proved uninhabitable by Europeans. As Chapters 2 and 3 explained,

---

[79] Robert Armstrong, *The Influence of Climate and Other Agents on the Human Constitution* (London: Longman, 1843), 106.

[80] Robert Lawson, 'Observations on the outbreak of yellow fever among the troops at Newcastle, Jamaica, in the latter part of 1856', *British Foreign Medical Review* 24 (1859), 324; *Naval and Military gazette*, 21 July 1838, 465.

[81] A. M. Tulloch, 'On the mortality among Her Majesty's troops serving in the colonies during the years 1844 and 1845', *Journal of the Statistical Society* 10 (1847), 252. The *United Service Journal*, looking back in 1864, attributed 'all the amelioration of the condition of the soldier that have since been affected' to Tulloch's recommendations. *United Service Journal* (1864), pt 2, 406.

[82] Ibid., 256–7.

those actually serving with the WIRs were continuously impressed by the physical capabilities of the men, including their stamina, strength and super-senses. In 1835 one physician had depicted the typical WIR soldier as 'a child of the sun, his physical adaption for warfare in a tropical climate is admirable in all respects'.[83] Tulloch, writing just three years later, believed that his data proved that black soldiers were not the superhuman soldiers some thought them to be. Almost ignoring the fact that European mortality rates were usually higher than those of the WIRs, he consistently stressed the unsuitability of black soldiers for service anywhere beyond their native African homelands. Previous military-medical authors had established that clear differences existed between the bodies of white and black soldiers. But what Tulloch had done was to take a largely positive interpretation of those differences and transform it into an entirely negative one. In the later 1840s and particularly in the 1850s, others would use Tulloch's statistics to try to prove, in an 'impartial' and 'scientific' manner, that black people differed in even more fundamental ways from white people and to such an extent that they could not be considered as members of a single human species.

---

[83] William Fergusson, 'On the qualities and employment of black troops in the West Indies', *United Service Journal* (1835), pt 1, 523.

5   Dehumanising the Black Soldier

Mid-nineteenth-century audiences in Britain, Europe and the United States voraciously consumed any published work based on voluminous statistics, and Alexander Tulloch's work on mortality in the British army had both encapsulated the zeitgeist and accelerated it. As Tulloch's publications began to be circulated to an ever-wider audience and reviewed in a variety of journals with a transatlantic reach, his conclusions about race and disease were picked up by one particularly important group of people: the 'American School' of ethnologists. Although numerous authors had written about what they perceived as key racial differences between Europeans, Africans and Asians over the previous century, the American School took it a stage further than most were willing to go. Key writers such as Samuel Morton and Josiah Nott argued that not only were Europeans physically and medically different from other races in important and widely accepted ways, they were so different as to constitute a separate and markedly superior species. Nott, in particular, would use these ideas to support pro-slavery arguments in the United States. These concepts did not go uncontested, but the statistics provided by Tulloch on comparative mortality were co-opted to support their ideas about the immutable biological differences between peoples. Anthropologists and physicians had drawn on an enormous variety of sources when debating human origins, including monumental inscriptions in Egypt, linguistics, the Bible, dissection and the detailed measurement of various body parts. Published medical statistics relating to the British army, and specifically the WIRs, became a significant, and arguably the most important, new piece of evidence that could be utilised.

Until the middle of the eighteenth century, the theory of climate had dominated thinking about human diversity. The earth clearly had a diversity of climate zones, such as frigid, temperate, torrid or desert, each inhabited by different varieties of humans. Put simply, people with the whitest skin were found in the coldest regions, while people with the darkest skin resided in the hottest.[1] Since climate was believed to cause human variation then, logically, as people moved from one climate to another, so their physicality should alter. This might not happen quickly, though white people could tan to quite a dark colour fairly rapidly, and indeed might take several generations to fully manifest itself. The problem by the middle of the eighteenth century was that Europeans had lived in tropical regions, such as the West Indies, Brazil and India, for a lengthy period, and none of them showed any imminent sign of developing physical features considered characteristic of black or brown people. Hair remained stubbornly straight, and if anything became lighter in the sun, while noses and lips remained comparatively petite. Similarly, Africans who had been transported throughout the Atlantic World, including Canada and northern Europe, had not developed European features or colouring even after many generations. The climate theory of human diversity was beginning to look increasingly frayed around the edges.

Several writers had challenged the theory of climate during the seventeenth and eighteenth centuries, suggesting instead that humans should more properly be divided into separate species. Naval surgeon John Atkins, after voyaging throughout the Atlantic World, was persuaded that 'the black and white race have, *ab origine*, sprung from different coloured first parents'.[2] One of the more prominent writers about race and slavery in the 1770s was Jamaican planter, administrator and legislator Edward Long. Long resided in Jamaica between 1757 and 1769, and his *History of Jamaica*, published in 1774 after his return to Britain, is the most detailed and comprehensive study of the island during the eighteenth century.[3] His comments about enslaved Africans reveal evidence of a man who probably thought more carefully about race than many contemporaries, and he certainly was not afraid to commit his most racist opinions to print. He speculated that

---

[1] Hannah Franziska Augustein (ed.), *Race: the Origins of an Idea, 1760–1850* (Bristol: Thoemmes Press, 1996), xiii.

[2] John Atkins, *A Voyage to Guinea, Brasil, and the West-Indies; in His Majesty's Ships, the Swallow and Weymouth* (London: Caesar Ward and Richard Chandler, 1735), 39. See also Suman Seth, *Difference and Disease: Medicine, Race and the Eighteenth-Century British Empire* (Cambridge: Cambridge University Press, 2018), 167–8; Colin Kidd, *The Forging of Races: Race and Scripture in the Protestant Atlantic World, 1600–2000* (Cambridge: Cambridge University Press, 2006), 118; Philip D. Curtin, *The Image of Africa: British Ideas and Action* (Madison: University of Wisconsin Press, 1964), 40–1. Seth points out that Atkins retreated from his polygenist views in later editions.

[3] See the online biography of Long at www.oxforddnb.com, as well as Curtin, *The Image of Africa*, 44–5; Seth, *Difference and Disease*, 208–40.

mulattoes might actually be infertile, and this was highly significant 'because it tends, among other evidences, to establish an opinion, which several have entertained, that the White and the Negro had not one common origin. … For my own part, I think there are extremely potent reasons for believing, that the White and the Negro are two distinct species'.[4] Warming to his theme, Long noted that the 'dark membrane which communicates that black colour to their skins, … does not alter by transportation into other climates', and in a wider critique of the theory of climate, he pointed out that Native Americans living on the same latitude as Africans did not have black skin.[5] It was more than black skin, of course, that marked Africans as different from other types of men. Long highlighted numerous other physical and intellectual traits where he thought the white race had proved itself superior to the black race. Africans were 'a brutish, ignorant, idle, crafty, treacherous, bloody, thievish, mistrustful, and superstitious people', totally 'void of genius' and an example of 'the vilest of the human kind, to which they have little more pretension of resemblance than what arises from their exterior form'. Indeed, Long spent two pages trying to claim that Africans and orangutans had more physical and cultural similarities than Africans and Europeans. Somewhat inevitably he concluded, 'When we reflect on the nature of these men, and their dissimilarity to the rest of mankind, must we not conclude, that they are a different species of the same genus?'[6]

Long's three volume *History of Jamaica* was published in London in 1774, and no doubt was of immediate interest to the absentee landowners who constituted the West India Committee of Merchants and Planters. It almost certainly came too late to influence Lord Henry Kames, a Scottish judge and enlightenment thinker whose *Sketches of the History of Man* was printed in Edinburgh the same year. Setting out to discover 'whether there be different races of men, or whether all men be of one race', Kames started from the position that as 'all men are not fitted equally for every climate', and because different climates evidently existed on earth, 'so there are different races of men fitted for these different climates'.[7] Yet this was not entirely satisfactory. Climate could not explain, as Long had also pointed out, why people in West and East Africa, or Central America, looked so different despite

---

[4] Edward Long, *The History of Jamaica* (London: T. Lowndes, 1774), II, 336.
[5] Ibid., 351–2.
[6] Ibid., 352–6, 359–60 (on orangutans).
[7] Henry Kames, *Sketches of the History of Man in Two Volumes* (Edinburgh: W. Creech, 1774), I, 1, 10–11.

experiencing similar tropical conditions. The only conclusion Kames could reach was that 'originally each kind was placed in its proper climate' – by God presumably.[8] Dismissing the objections of those who defined a species as capable of producing fertile offspring, which men and women from every part of the globe were clearly able to do, Kames noted that there were several examples of different animal species that occasionally interbred successfully. In contrast to Long and many later writers, Kames was not entirely derogatory in his description of non-whites. Although he initially believed that 'inferiority in their under-standing' supported his case that black people were a different species to whites, 'upon second thoughts' he wondered if it was 'occasioned by their condition'. The natives of the Gold Coast, he had heard, 'are industrious, apprehend readily what is said to them, have a good judge-ment, [and] are equitable in their dealings'.[9]

Although widely read, Kames's *Sketches* for instance was reprinted in Dublin, London and Philadelphia and a revised second edition appeared in 1788, Long and Kames were unable to change the overall tenor of the debate about human origins. Colin Kidd has argued that the reception among the scientific community to their nascent polygen-ism was in fact 'roundly hostile'.[10] The argument for polygenesis they put forward found numerous critics among clergymen outraged at a ver-sion of creation so completely at odds with the one outlined in the Bible. Presbyterian Samuel Stanhope Smith, later president of Princeton, was among the first to challenge the easy dismissal of climate as the main cause of bodily differences in people. In his 1787 *Essay on the Causes of the Variety of Complexion and Figure in the Human Species*, which some historians have seen as the 'most important and influential American statement of monogenism', Smith argued that long exposure to the heat of the sun over generations was more than sufficient to turn Africans black, particularly when compared with just how tanned a white person could become if they worked outside all their life.[11] He believed that black people in the northern states of the United States tended to be lighter than their brethren in the southern states, proof, he thought, that climate was fully capable of exerting a significant influence over

---

[8] Ibid. I, 38. God also was granted a role by Long, who argued that he believed human variety 'to form the same gradual climax towards perfection in this human system, which is so evidently designed in every other'. Long, *History of Jamaica*, II, 371.

[9] Kames, *Sketches of the History of Man*, I, 32.

[10] Kidd, *Forging of Races*, 102.

[11] Bruce Dain, *A Hideous Monster of the Mind: American Race Theory in the Early Republic* (Cambridge and London: Harvard University Press, 2002), 41.

human bodies.[12] As for Kames's claim that 'men, by making great and sudden changes of climate or country, are exposed to disease' and thus were proven to be naturally unsuited to other climates, Smith had an easy answer: changes should be gradual to allow time for the body to assimilate and adjust since 'experience teaches us that mankind can exist in every climate'.[13] This was a reaffirmation of the belief that the seasoning process proved human unity. British physician James Cowles Prichard agreed with Smith that while there were clearly great differences between the different races of men, these were essentially superficial and did not mean that different human species existed. The first edition of his widely read and cited *Researches into the Physical History of Man*, published in 1813, went so far as to speculate that the 'primitive stock of men were probably Negroes', and he wondered if evidence might be found to show 'that the fairest races of white people in Europe, are descended from, or have any affinity with Negroes'.[14]

Even though Long and Kames failed to gain a widespread acceptance of their polygenist ideas in the 1780s and 1790s, a few determined adherents thought they had actually articulated a new truth about the origins of man. Focussing just on Africans and Europeans, Dr Charles White outlined what he considered to be the major differences between the races: Africans had a skeleton that 'approached the ape' and had thicker skin; they sweated less but emitted a 'rank smell'; and they 'seem[ed] to suffer more than we do from cold'.[15] Significantly White co-opted an argument first made by Frederick Blumenbach that highlighted differential responses to disease as a key marker of difference between species.[16] If all men belonged to just one species, then the impact of disease would be broadly similar. White saw this as a weakness in the argument for human unity, noting that the fabled immunity

---

[12] Samuel Stanhope Smith, *Essay on the Causes of the Variety of Complexion and Figure in the Human Species* (Philadelphia: Robert Aitken, 1787), 11; David N. Livingstone, *Adam's Ancestors: Race, Religion and the Politics of Human Origins* (Baltimore: Johns Hopkins University Press, 2008), 74–5.

[13] Smith, *Essay on the Causes of the Variety*, Appendix 2, 22.

[14] James Cowles Prichard, *Researches into the Physical History of Man* (London: John and Arthur Arch, 1813), 238–9. Brent Henze, 'Scientific definition in rhetorical formations: race as "permanent variety" in James Cowles Prichard's ethnology', *Rhetoric Review* 23 (2004), 323. See also 'Account of a paper read by before the Royal Society by Dr Wells', in the *London Medical and Physical Journal* 29 (1813), 508. Wells believed that given sufficient generations, white people would gradually transform into black people in the tropics.

[15] Charles White, *An Account of the Regular Gradation in Man* (London: C. Dilly, 1799), 43, 58–9.

[16] Augustein, ed., *Race*, xvii.

of Africans to tropical fevers was balanced by greater susceptibility to other illnesses. His main sources for this claim were published works by British army physicians such as Benjamin Moseley and John Hunter, men who had worked alongside, and treated, black soldiers. As to the fertility of hybrids, White repeated Long's assertion (but without providing any additional supporting evidence) that 'he never knew two mulattoes to have any offspring'.[17]

In general, however, those writing about the history of human beings in the early years of the nineteenth century were more likely to follow Prichard and see all of humanity as a single species, only varied by climate. John Bigland, writing in 1816, argued that 'the African, and southern Asiatic, under the influence of an ardent sun, are fiery, sensual, and vindictive' and that climate had a 'very powerful influence on the corporeal frame of man'. Such was the unremitting influence of climate that the changes wrought by the sun were, he believed, 'transmissible by hereditary descent'.[18] That is not to say that differences between Europeans and other peoples were overlooked, indeed most writers were happy to affirm the superiority of European technology, civilisation and culture over all other peoples. William Lawrence agreed with White that 'the Negro is more like a monkey than the European', but crucially that did not actually make him an ape. Rather 'the negro and the European are the two extremities of a very long gradation; between them are almost innumerable intermediate states which differ from each other no more than the individuals occasionally produced in every race differ from the generality of the race'.[19] As proof of the existence of this gradation, Lawrence pointed to mulattoes, claiming they were half way between white and black, while 'in cleanliness, capacity, activity, and courage, they are decidedly superior to the Negroes'.[20]

By the 1830s intellectual currents had begun to shift in favour of polygenesis, aided by the rise of new sciences such as phrenology.[21] George Combe believed the skulls owned by the Edinburgh Phrenology Society (founded in 1820) proved that everyone 'obviously inherits from

---

[17] White, *An Account of the Regular Gradation in Man*, 73–80, 129–30.
[18] John Bigland, *Historical Display of the Effects of Physical and Moral Causes on the Character and Circumstances of Nations* (London: Longman, 1816), 13, 18, 89.
[19] William Lawrence, *Lectures on Physiology, Zoology, and the Natural History of Man* (London: J. Callow, 1819), 125, 304.
[20] Ibid., 295.
[21] Philip Curtin and Nancy Stepan have both pointed out that this was 'science at its best for the time' and therefore we should avoid viewing it with a modern-day lens. Curtin, *The Image of Africa*, 29; Nancy Stepan, *The Idea of Race in Science* (London: Macmillan, 1982), xvi.

his parents a certain general type of head', and that as a result science should talk about 'national brains' as much as 'national character'.[22] The shift in thought patterns can be discerned in the *Medico Chirurgical Review*. In 1829 the *MCR* had reaffirmed faith in 'the instrumentality of climate' as the key factor causing human 'physical peculiarities'. Just four years later it was the other way around, with the blood, skin and hair of Africans naturally 'fitting him for the vertical sun of Africa'. Moreover, the 'difference of conformation' between the skulls of Europeans and Africans confirmed that they would never 'by the utmost stretch of human ingenuity' be intellectual equals.[23]

Colin Kidd has argued that the struggle between monogenesis and polygenesis should be seen as part of a wider 'crisis of faith' in the nineteenth century.[24] Advocates for polygenesis knew that overcoming the opposition of religiously minded individuals, who adhered to the single creation described in Genesis, was one of their biggest tasks. Some embraced the challenge willingly and directly. Critical of mindless 'dogma' that rejected new evidence, Kentucky physician Charles Caldwell consigned the Bible to 'moral and religious instruction' with 'no authority in physical science'.[25] For one thing, the Bible's own internal chronology worked against the idea of human unity. Scholars had established a set date for creation and the other events described in Genesis, but historians and archaeologists had proved that dark-skinned Ethiopians had existed for a similar amount of time, and unless these men had somehow transmuted from white to black, or vice versa, in a very short space of time, then they had to have been created separately. This was not to deny God a role. Polygenesis asserted the idea of multiple creations, all by God, with the book of Genesis only describing that of the white man. Caldwell then listed all the superficial physical differences between white and black people, including skin, hair and skull shape, before moving on to internal differences. The fact that 'it is known to everyone, that, in tropical climates, the African race enjoys much better health than the Caucasian' Caldwell explained by claiming that Africans had a more adaptive liver.[26] And who else but God would have placed Africans in an environment 'where they enjoy

---

[22] George Combe, *The Constitution of Man* (Edinburgh: John Anderson, 1828, Cambridge University Press reprint, 2009), 145–6.

[23] *Medico Chirurgical Review*, 11 (1829), 121; 19 (1833), 151.

[24] Kidd, *Forging of Races*, 121–68.

[25] Charles Caldwell, *Thoughts on the Original Unity of the Human Race* (New York: E. Bliss, 1830), 15.

[26] Ibid., 112. One of the authors Caldwell had read was John Hunter; see p. 41 of Caldwell's *Thoughts*.

most health, live to the greatest age, and attain the highest perfection of their nature'. Thus the 'privileges and favours conferred by their Creator' ensured that Africans in Africa would 'be healthy and happy, vigorous and fruitful from the beginning'. By contrast white people in Africa quickly succumbed to 'sickness, mortality, and great degeneracy in strength'.[27] Accepting polygenesis was, in this sense, simply acknowledging the natural order of the world.

The degree of susceptibility to disease now began to take centre stage in the argument between the monogenists and polygenists, and it would be in this field that the writings and data relating to the WIRs would end up being used by the polygenists in some of their most telling contributions. In the 1826 second edition of *Researches into the Physical History of Man*, James Prichard sought to bolster his argument that humans were a single species by highlighting the uniform action of disease. He argued that 'contagious diseases which belong to the human kind, are very nearly, if not without any exception whatever, confined to it, and quite incapable of producing in the lower animals an analogous disease'.[28] Humans, according to Prichard, did not catch illness from animals, nor vice versa. On the other hand, he asserted it as 'an undoubted fact, that all human contagious, and all epidemic diseases, are capable of exerting their pernicious influence on all the tribes of men', though he was prepared to concede, given the sheer weight of evidence, that 'the natives of particular climates suffer more than others'.[29] For Prichard this was not a binary choice, rather one of degree. The third edition of his work, published in 1837, was even more categorical – there was no disease 'which is peculiar to one race, or incapable of attacking others', and the most he would accept was that 'the predisposition to any given disease is different in different races'.[30] Opponents such as Caldwell scoffed at Prichard's research, pointing to plenty of diseases that afflicted humans and animals alike, including 'scrofula, measles and influenza'. Since Prichard accepted the principle of variable susceptibility to disease, surely it was more logical to suppose that people had been specifically created to inhabit different climates, rather than forcing them to endure 'centuries of sickness and misery' as they adapted.[31] Some authors tried to tread a rather confused middle course

---

[27] Ibid., 158–9.
[28] James Cowles Prichard, *Researches in the Physical History of Man*, 2nd ed. (London: J. McCreary, 1826), I, 120.
[29] Ibid., 121.
[30] James Cowles Prichard, *Researches into the Physical History of Man*, 3rd ed. (London: Sherwood, Gilbert and Piper, 1837), II, 152.
[31] Caldwell, *Thoughts on the Original Unity of the Human Race*, 133, 164.

between the two extremes. W. C. Linnaeus Martin accepted that it was an issue of 'great difficulty', but as there were 'no natural causes' he could think of that would change a white man into a black one, he agreed with the polygenists that men had been 'formed *for* the regions they inhabit, and not *by* them'. At the same time, and even on the same page, he agreed with the monogenists that black people 'are of the same species with the other families of mankind'.[32] Other writers said little about the origins of humanity *per se* but drew conclusions that could be used to support the polygenist argument. Richard Reece's *The Medical Guide for Tropical Climates* was just one of the numerous medical self-help texts he published. He observed that due to a 'particular habit of body' there were several tropical diseases that only afflicted white people, while different diseases honed in on black bodies.[33] And this was particularly obvious to those dwelling in the tropics. John Stewart, a long-time resident of Jamaica, recorded that in his experience black and white people were indeed susceptible to different illnesses, so much so in fact that it was 'as if the bodily system, as well as habits of the two races, were of an opposite nature'.[34] The contrast with the beliefs of most eighteenth-century West Indian physicians, outlined in the intro-duction, could not be more stark.

Some physicians followed Caldwell's lead and began to advocate different medical treatments for different races based on the idea that diseases were 'modified by the peculiarities which attach to the dif-ferent varieties of man'. Kentucky doctor Lunsford Vandell argued that because of the innate hereditary differences, including thicker skin and the 'undue development' of cellular tissue, black people were more prone to tetanus and scrofula, but less liable to cholera and most forms of fever.[35] French doctor Julien-Joseph Virey had published his *Histoire naturelle du genre humain* in 1801, with a second edition in 1824. Parts of the work were translated into English and published as the *Natural History of the Negro Race* in 1837. Virey believed that 'several diseases of the negro, are quite different from those of the

---

[32] W. C. Linnaeus Martin, *A General Introduction to the Natural History of Mammiferous Animals* (London: Wright and Co., 1841), 167–9.

[33] Richard Reece, *The Medical Guide for Tropical Climates* (London: Longman, Hurst, Reese, Orme and Brown, 1814), 171.

[34] J. Stewart, *A View of the Past and Present State of the Island of Jamaica: with Remarks on the Moral and Physical Condition of the Slaves and the Abolition of Slavery in the Colonies* (Edinburgh: Oliver and Boyd, 1823), 307.

[35] Lunsford P. Vandell, 'Remarks on struma Africana, or the disease usually called negro poison or negro consumption', *Transylvania Journal of Medicine and Associate Sciences* 4 (1831), 91.

white man', and since 'contagious diseases which affect a species, are not communicated to another even the next to it, because there is a difference in their constitutions, in like manner, white men living with negroes are not liable to the Pian, a disease very contagious among the blacks'.[36] His compatriot J. M. A. Goupil, attached to the military hospital in Toulouse, similarly believed that 'the impression of cold air on a negro child is sufficient to produce tetanus, while it would rarely be produced by the same causes in the inhabitants of Russia'.[37] Goupil's work was published in Paris in 1824, and translated by Josiah Nott for the American audience in 1831.

Physicians and anthropologists alike were edging ever closer to accepting that white and black bodies were fundamentally and innately different, something that WIR surgeons had been saying for a while. But it was the new science of ethnology that would turbocharge the idea and propel it into the intellectual mainstream. Ethnology had plenty of adherents in Europe, but it was in the United States that it would find its most eloquent advocates. The leading figure of the American School of ethnology was Philadelphia physician Samuel Morton. Morton's importance in the field lies not so much in his creation of 'the idea that human diversity had a biological basis and could not be altered' but in its wide dissemination.[38] Morton expended considerable energy in collecting skulls from all over the world and then measuring their capacity in his quest to prove that humanity was divided into several species. His results, showing that Europeans had larger skulls and thus larger brains than those of African or Asian origin, handily ignored the work of other scientists on skull capacities that had produced markedly different results. Frederick Tiedemann's research, as presented to the Royal Society in 1836 for example, found 'no perceptible difference exists either in the average weight or the average size of the brain of the Negro and of the European'.[39] Morton's *Crania Americana* (1839) and *Crania Aegyptiaca* (1844) gained a wide circulation, and elevated him to the role of father figure in the American School of ethnology, but he actually said very little about comparative disease resistance in his published works. The most he was prepared to say on the matter was to claim that the obvious and well-known affinity of Africans for

---

[36] J.-J. Virey, *Natural History of the Negro Race* (J. H. Guenebault, trans.) (Charleston: D. J. Dowling, 1837), 76–7.
[37] J. M. A. Goupil, *An Exposition on the Principles of the New Medical Doctrine* (J. Nott, trans.) (Columbia: Times and Gazette Office, 1831), 70.
[38] Dain, *Hideous Monster*, 198, 217–18. Stephen Jay Gould, *The Mismeasure of Man* (New York: Norton, 1996), 82–104.
[39] *British and Foreign Medical Review* 4 (1837), 530.

hot tropical climates, places where 'the European constitution at once becomes the victim of enervating and destroying fevers', proved that there was 'a primeval difference among men'.[40]

The man who would follow Morton's lead, and become the standard bearer for the American polygenists, was Josiah Nott, a doctor residing in Mobile, Alabama.[41] In his earliest publications Nott was cautious in his approach to the idea of polygenesis. Although much of his argument in 'The mulatto a hybrid' (1843), wherein he follows Long's work from seventy years earlier by claiming that mulattoes are 'bad breeders...many of them do not conceive at all', clearly lent credence to those who believed whites and blacks to be different species, Nott was actually more reticent. The different races, he wrote, 'may have been distinct creations or may be mere varieties of the same species, produced by external causes acting through many thousand years'.[42] Just a year later Nott had become distinctly more fixed in his view and, crucially, he used the argument that had been put forward by Tulloch on extreme local adaptability to make his case. Each race of man, claimed Nott, had a climate to which he was adapted, and none could safely relocate from their original climate. Thus 'the black man was placed in tropical Africa, because he was suited to this climate and no other'.[43] When Africans were taken out of Africa and brought to the United States, they fared less well the further north they went, and in Philadelphia, where Nott had worked for a time at the alms-house, he claimed it was well-known among local physicians that black residents 'suffered more than the whites from diseases of cold'.[44] Indeed such was the inability of black people to endure cold that Nott suggested they 'would become extinct in New England, if cut off from immigration'.[45] In the southern states the opposite was true: black people coped better

[40] Samuel Morton, *Brief Remarks on the Diversities of the Human Species* (Philadelphia: Merrihew and Thompson, 1842), 9, 6.

[41] For an overview of Nott's career as an ethnologist, see C. Loring Brace, 'The "ethnology" of Josiah Clark Nott', *Bulletin of the New York Academy of Medicine* 50 (1974), 509–28; Paul Erickson, 'The anthropology of Josiah Clark Nott', *Kroeber Anthropological Society Papers* 65–66 (1986), 103–20. The best biography of Nott remains Reginald Horsman, *Josiah Nott of Mobile: Southerner, Physician, and Racial Theorist* (Baton Rouge: Louisiana State University Press, 1987). See also Kidd, *Forging of Races*, 144–5.

[42] Josiah Nott, 'The mulatto a hybrid', *Boston Medical and Surgical Journal* 29 (1843), 29–30.

[43] Josiah Nott, *Two Lectures on the Natural History of the Caucasian and Negro Races* (Mobile: Dade and Thompson, 1844), 29.

[44] Josiah Nott, 'Unity of the human race', *Southern Quarterly Review* 9 (1846), 17. See also James Thomson, *A Treatise on the Diseases of Negroes as They Occur in the Island of Jamaica* (Jamaica: Alex Aikman, 1820), 7.

[45] J. C. Nott, 'Geographical distribution of animals and the races of men', *New Orleans Medical and Surgical Journal* 9 (1852), 733.

in the hot climate than whites and were immune to illness like malaria and yellow fever. In Nott's opinion the climate of the South was evidently close enough to West Africa to give black people a comparative advantage. Indeed, in the case of yellow fever, the innate protection Nott perceived among blacks was something that he thought must be contained in 'negro blood' since 'the smallest admixture of it with the white will protect against this disease'.[46] And if immunity to fever was inheritable via blood, then it was clearly something that the enslaved population of the South could thank their African ancestors for.

As a long-time resident of Mobile, Alabama, Nott had witnessed the impact of yellow fever epidemics first-hand. As the population of the city grew so did the death toll, rising from approximately 450 in the 1839 epidemic to more than 1,000 in 1853. Mobile's epidemics often coincided with outbreaks in nearby New Orleans, as the two ports were well connected by ship. Nott was perfectly aware from personal observation that yellow fever was a discriminating disease, attacking certain classes of residents while leaving others untouched. The most significant factor, he insisted, was race: 'During the severe epidemics of yellow of fever in Mobile in the years 1837, '39 and '42 I did not see a single individual attacked with this disease, who was in the remotest degree allied to the Negro race'.[47] Nott was being hugely disingenuous of course. He would have known perfectly well that residency determined vulnerability to yellow fever, with long-time residents (white or black) surviving a previous infection being immune while newly arrived working-class whites, often from Ireland, possessed no immunity and succumbed in droves. It suited him, however, to highlight racial immunity. Despite his deliberate obfuscation, Nott actually came closer than most physicians to discovering that yellow fever is transmitted by mosquitoes. His 1848 article 'Yellow fever contrasted with bilious fever' was based on the hypothesis that 'some form of insect life' was responsible, pointing to the fact that a killing frost, known to stop yellow fever in its tracks, would destroy 'insects and their eggs' but have little effect on 'miasmas' or other popular explanations for the disease. He even specifically mentioned 'some insect or animalcule, hatched in the lowlands, like the musquito' as a possible agent, but unfortunately his ideas did not gain much traction and it would be the twentieth century before the link between mosquitoes and tropical diseases was proven beyond doubt.[48]

---

[46] Josiah Nott, 'Statistics of southern slave populations', *De Bow's Commercial Review of the South and West* 2 (1847), 281.

[47] Nott, 'The mulatto a hybrid', 30.

[48] J. C. Nott, 'Yellow fever contrasted with bilious fever', *New Orleans Medical and Surgical Journal* 4 (1848), 563, 580.

Nott's work on yellow fever has tended to be overlooked, both by contemporaries and later historians, who focus on his more popular polygenist publications, but it is important because in researching the disease he consumed numerous publications by British military surgeons.[49] Among those he cited were John Pringle, whose influential *Observations on the Diseases of the Army in Camp and Garrison* (1750) was one of the first to propose changes, including an improved diet, better accommodation and medical care, to reduce military mortality; James Johnston, author of *The Influence of Tropical Climates on European Constitutions* (1812) and founder of the *Medico Chirurgical Journal*; and William Fergusson, whose *Inquiry into Yellow Fever* (1817) had been prompted by his service alongside members of the WIRs in the Caribbean. Nott's argument that even a small amount of black blood could grant immunity to tropical fevers was probably influenced by the work of William Wright, who served in St Domingue before assuming command of the main hospital in Barbados. Wright claimed there was a significant difference between the blood of sick black people, 'generally firm and often buffy', and that of sick white people, 'loose, discoloured and watery'. It was clearly sufficiently different, he thought, to affect susceptibility to illnesses.[50] The publications of Robert Jackson, who served in the West Indies and eventually rose to be inspector of army hospitals, proved to be particularly useful to Nott. Jackson's *Treatise on the Fevers of Jamaica* (1791) supported the idea that native Africans were immune to yellow fever; his *Outline of the History and Cure of Fever* (1798) singled out Africans who 'have experienced frequent changes of climate' as being particularly vulnerable to diseases; while the *Systematic View of the Formation, Discipline and Economy of Armies* (1804) claimed that mulattoes were 'neither hardy nor strong in body', a claim that Nott had repeated and extended in his first publication in 1843.[51] Nott would return to these and other British military authors as he refined his polygenist ideas.

---

[49] Exceptions are W. G. Downs, 'Yellow fever and Josiah Clark Nott', *Bulletin of the New York Academy of Medicine* 50 (1974), 499–508, and Eli Chernin, 'Josiah Clark Nott, insects, and yellow fever', *Bulletin of the New York Academy of Medicine* 59 (1983), 790–802.

[50] William Wright, *Memoir of the Late William Wright* (Edinburgh: William Blackwood 1828), 407.

[51] Robert Jackson, *A Treatise on the Fevers of Jamaica, with Some Observations on the Intermitting Fever of America* (London: J. Murray, 1791), 249; Robert Jackson, *An Outline of the History and Cure of Fever, Endemic and Contagious* (Edinburgh: Mundell and Son, 1798), 328; Robert Jackson, *A Systematic View of the Formation, Discipline and Economy of Armies* (London: John Stockdale, 1804), 9.

Nott's two major interventions in the debate about the origins of man were his *Types of Mankind: or, Ethnological Researches: Based upon the Ancient Monuments, Paintings, Sculptures, and Crania of Races, and upon Their Natural, Geographical, Philological and Biblical History* (1854) and *Indigenous Races of the Earth; or, New Chapters of Ethnological Inquiry; Including Monographs on Special Departments* (1857), both co-authored with George Gliddon. The two volumes were the culmination of several years of reflection on the issue, and there is no doubt that Nott set out to be deliberately provocative at times. In September 1848 he wrote to a friend that he had received an invitation to give a lecture on 'Niggerology' in New Orleans, something he expected to provide 'rare sport'.[52] Publishing a version of the lectures in 1849 would, he knew, 'stir up hell in the *Christians* and bring down a shower of fire and brimstone on me before long' but that did not bother him. Although in print Nott was willing to afford 'full respect' to those with 'religious convictions', in private he was cynical about theology: 'religion you know is a funny thing, a man's conscience is always on the side of his interest'.[53] Nott professed that his main purpose in publishing his thoughts on the origins of man was to 'assist in developing the truths involved in the discussion', though he confided to a friend, 'My experience has taught me that if a man wants to get on fast he must kick up a dam'd fuss', and without something of a 'notoriety... the tide will run by them'.[54] His two major publications on the topic, *Types of Mankind* and *Indigenous Races of the Earth* certainly did 'kick up a dam'd fuss'.

Types of Mankind reiterates many of the claims Nott had made in his earlier writings, for example, that immunity to tropical illnesses was conferred by even a 'small trace of negro blood'. The book was hugely popular, selling out a print run of 3,500 within four months and being reprinted several times.[55] *Indigenous Races* goes further, particularly in

---

[52] Nott to Squier, 30 September 1848. E. G. Squier Papers, Library of Congress (microfilm).

[53] Josiah C. Nott, *An Essay on the Natural History of Mankind Viewed in Connection with Negro Slavery* (Mobile: Dade, Thompson and Co., 1851), 9; Nott to Squier, 9 August 1849; E. G. Squier Papers, Library of Congress.

[54] Nott to Squier, 30 April 1854 and 2 March 1850, E. G. Squier Papers, Library of Congress.

[55] J. C. Nott and George R. Gliddon, *Types of Mankind* (Philadelphia: Lippincott, Grambo and Co., 1854), 68; Dain, *Hideous Monster*, 225. According to one historian it became 'the most widely read work on polygenism'. B. Riccardo Brown, *Until Darwin: Science, Human Variety and the Origins of Race* (London: Pickering and Chatto, 2010), 90.

the discussion of the relationships among race, climate and disease. Starting out from the presumption that 'the white and black races ... are distinct species ... if we can show that these races are not affected in like manner by diseases, we fortify the conclusion to which natural history has led us'. Nott argued that 'as long as a race preserves its peculiar physiological structure and laws, it must to some extent be peculiarly affected by morbific influences'.[56] Drawing on his own personal experience, that of other US physicians and published US mortality statistics, Nott listed a wide variety of illness that impacted blacks more than whites, particularly related to the 'acute diseases of winter'. Official mortality statistics showed that 'the mortality of blacks in our Northern States averages about double that of the whites', and even in the South where the winter was far milder, the patients in Nott's own 'private infirmary, devoted to negroes' suffered more in the winter than the summer. He recommended that treatment regimens should be determined by race. Blood-letting, a staple treatment for most white patients, was often ruled out for black patients and instead 'stimulants' were prescribed – intended to have the exact opposite effect of blood-letting.[57] For Nott, the evidence clearly supported his claim that disease impacted blacks and whites differently.

Aware that some might dispute his conclusions and point to his residence in a slaveholding state as an indicator of bias, Nott sought validation of his argument in impartial sources, ones that could not be seen as tainted by slavery. Nott read widely, in several languages, and eagerly sought books and periodicals from overseas. In an 1848 letter to a friend, Nott reported that 'I have a good deal of rich material on hand and [am] expecting a considerable addition of rich and rare books from Europe in a few days'. In other letters he mentioned subscribing to British periodicals, and that he had to 'send abroad for all my books'.[58] The obvious place to turn for evidence confirming his argument were the publications of the British military. Britain had abolished slavery and its replacement – apprenticeship – by 1838, and actively patrolled the oceans suppressing the slave trade. It could hardly be accused of supporting slavery as an institution. At the same time the British Empire was vast, and the army had regular contact with a wide variety of peoples. The numerous publications of the army,

---

[56] J. C. Nott and George R. Gliddon, *Indigenous Races of the Earth* (Philadelphia: Lippincott and Co., 1857), 360, 362.
[57] Ibid., 368.
[58] Nott to Squier, 19 August 1848 and 2 March 1850, E. G. Squier Papers, Library of Congress.

particularly those of army physicians, attracted Nott's attention, especially when they seemingly confirmed his argument. On the inability of Europeans to acclimatise to tropical conditions, he noted that 'the English army surgeons tell us that Englishmen do not become acclimated in India; length of residence affords no immunity, but, on the contrary, the mortality among officers and troops is greatest among those who would remain longest in the climate'.[59] This was precisely the argument that Tulloch had made regarding what he called the 'myth' of acclimation in the West Indies in 1838. And it was from Tulloch's published volumes, or at least the extensive reviews of them published in American periodicals, that Nott would find the greatest evidence to support his case that black and white people were susceptible to different diseases.

Without access to Tulloch's original four printed volumes, which traversed the Atlantic in very limited numbers, Nott relied on the review of the volume covering Africa, including lengthy passages copied verbatim, published in the *Medico Chirurgical Review* in April 1840. Tulloch's data, according to Nott, provided 'the most minute and reliable statistics we possess, touching the influence of tropical climates on the European races'. Here was irrefutable evidence, he claimed, of the permanence of differential racial vulnerability to disease. The experience of the 2WIR in Sierra Leone in 1825 clearly illustrated Nott's point. As was entirely predictable, most of the 300 white troops attached to the 2WIR quickly sickened and died of tropical illnesses, whereas the 2WIR 'only lost one man, and had seldom any in the hospital'. What was significant to Nott was that the men of the 2WIR 'had been born and brought up in the West Indies; and, according to the commonly received theory of acclimation, should not have enjoyed this exemption'. These men were proof, he thought, that they had inherited specific disease resistance from their African forebears, something that no white men could ever acquire. Indeed, given Tulloch's assault on the very idea of seasoning, Nott went so far as to claim that 'no length of residence acclimated the whites in Africa; on the contrary, it exterminates them'.[60] Of course significant holes can be poked into Nott's discussion of Tulloch's statistics. For one thing, the vast majority of the 2WIR serving in Sierra Leone in 1825 had been born in Africa, not the West Indies, and therefore would probably have acquired immunity to endemic West African diseases, such as yellow fever, as children.[61] Nott would not necessarily

[59] Nott and Gliddon, *Indigenous Races of the Earth*, 365.
[60] Ibid., 374–5.
[61] See the 2WIR Regimental succession books, WO 25/644-645.

have been aware of this, since the army's recruiting tactics in Sierra Leone were not widely publicised.

Nott next took up Tulloch's 1847 article, published in the *Journal of Statistical Society of London*, which he evidently had to hand. The article, 'On the mortality among Her Majesty's troops serving in the colonies during the years 1844 and 1845', was essentially a brief update on the four volumes that Tulloch had published between 1838 and 1841. Quoting a large section of the article verbatim, Nott seized on Tulloch's conclusion that soldiers could never become truly assimilated to lands beyond their native homeland. By claiming that the statistics 'point out the limits intended by nature for particular races: and within which alone they can thrive and increase', Tulloch had, perhaps unwittingly, provided grist to Nott's mill. Lauding Tulloch's data, 'which are remarkable for their fullness and the unprejudiced tone in which they are given', Nott was able to claim that 'certain races cannot become assimilated to certain climates... [and] the negro, in most regions out of Africa, whether within the Tropics – as in the Antilles, or out of them – as at Gibraltar, is gradually exterminated'.[62] The United States remained a glaring exception to this rule, of course, with the enslaved population continuing to grow, a point that Nott usually overlooked.

Nott was not the only polygenist to make use of the publications of British military surgeons; indeed the works of John Hunter, Colin Chisholm, William Fergusson and many others featured prominently in American medical journals. Dr W. G. Ramsay used Benjamin Moseley's *Treatise on Tropical Climates* (1789) to support his own argument that 'the sensibility of the negro is much less acute than that of the European, the former enduring pain with less apparent suffering that the latter'. And given the well-established exemption of black people to 'febrile disorders' because 'their skin is so well adapted to the climate in which they live', as well as their greater susceptibility to typhus and their inability to 'bear depleting remedies as well as whites', it was clear, he concluded, that 'the stories propagated by a few and credited by many of their approximation to the Europeans, are perfectly groundless'.[63] Scottish surgeon Robert Knox had actually seen active service in South Africa between 1817 and 1820, but his *Races of Men* (1850) drew on a variety of other military writers, including Hector M'Lean's 1797 study

---

[62] Nott and Gliddon, *Indigenous Races of the Earth*, 386.
[63] W. G. Ramsay, 'The physiological differences between the European (or white man) and the negro', *Southern Agriculturalist* 12 (1839), 412–18. See also Martin S. Pernick, *A Calculus of Suffering: Pain, Professionalism, and Anesthesia in Nineteenth-Century America* (New York: Columbia University Press, 1985), 154.

of troop mortality in Haiti and James Tuckey's 1818 account of an expedition to the Congo, as well as Tulloch's volumes of medical statistics. These works provided, claimed Knox, 'unanswerable proof against the possibility of colonizing a tropical country with European men' since whenever Europeans ventured into the tropics only death awaited them. Each race was consigned 'to those quarters of the earth which Nature seems to have assigned it'.[64] Dr R. La Roche used not only Tulloch's data but also the writings of William Fergusson and Robert Jackson to confirm 'that blacks are much less liable than whites to other forms of miasmal fevers, and that when attacked, they have the disease in a milder form' and that this applied even when compared with whites who had been born in a tropical climate. Conversely, pneumonia was 'the most common form of disease that occurs among the transplanted natives of Africa, whether such as are enrolled in the lists of the army, or such as are reserved for field labour'.[65]

Even Charles Darwin was intrigued by the publications of army surgeons relating to comparative immunity. The work of William Fergusson in particular caused Darwin to muse whether the immunity of black people to tropical fevers might be 'something to do with the skin's texture' and if 'the ideosyncracy of the Negro (and partly mulatto) prevents his taking any form of Malaria', then naturalists might consider this to be an 'adaptation and Species-like'. Ultimately Darwin's own most significant publications *On the Origin of Species* (1859) and *The Descent of Man* (1871) determined that it was not 'species-like' at all, and he would ultimately demolish the idea of any kind of 'genesis'.[66]

Frenchman Jean Boudin, chief physician to the army of the Alps and 'leading authority in military medicine', also made extensive use of British military statistics in his *Études de pathologie comparée* (1847). While there

---

[64] Robert Knox, *The Races of Men: a Fragment* (Philadelphia: Lea and Blanchard, 1850), 193–4. The works referenced were Hector M'Lean, *An Enquiry into the Nature and Causes of the Great Mortality among the Troops at St Domingo* (London: T. Cadell, 1797), and James Hingston Tuckey, *Narrative of an Expedition to Explore the River Zaire, Usually Called the Congo, in South Africa, in 1816* (London: J. Murray, 1818). On Knox, see also Evelleen Richards, 'The "moral anatomy" of Robert Knox: the interplay between biological and social thought in Victorian scientific naturalism', *Journal of the History of Biology* 22 (1989), 373–436.

[65] R. La Roche, 'Remarks on the connection, pathological and etiological, supposed to exist between pneumonia and periodic fever', *Charleston Medical Journal* 8 (1853), 578, 582.

[66] Charles Darwin, *On the Origin of Species by Means of Natural Selection* (London: John Murray, 1859); Darwin, *The Descent of Man and Selection in Relation to Sex* (London: John Murray, 1871). Adrian Desmond and James Moore, *Darwin's Sacred Cause: Race, Slavery and the Quest for Human Origins* (London: Allen Lane, 2009), 129–30; Edward Beasley, 'Making Races', *Victorian Review* 40 (2014), 50.

was no English edition of his book, it was reviewed in English language periodicals, and American polygenists seized on his work as providing another 'impartial' voice to support their cause. Boudin's study of medical statistics gathered on French troops stationed in Algeria convinced him that Europeans could 'not become inured to the climate by long residence'. In the same manner, the volumes published by Tulloch were used and cited by Boudin as proving that 'the most trifling losses are experienced in general by troops serving in their native country.... The inverse takes place with negro troops, among whom mortality increases obviously in the direct ratio of their removal from the tropics'.[67] Describing him as the 'distinguished military physician', Nott made extensive use of Boudin's published works, personally mailed to him by the author, and was gratified to read confirmation 'of all our assertions with regard to the comparative exemption of negroes from malarial diseases, and their greater liability to typhoid and lung diseases, as well as cholera'.[68] Examples of black troops failing to adapt to colder climates abounded. Boudin claimed the 4WIR in Gibraltar had been 'almost entirely destroyed by pulmonary consumption' within two years, while black soldiers in Ceylon had suffered terribly when garrisoning mountain outposts.[69]

In the 1840s and 1850s, Boudin was just one of several authors to re-examine the experiences of the 4WIR in Gibraltar. Tulloch had used the data from the 4WIR between 1817 and 1819 to prove his case that black troops were unsuitable for service, on medical grounds, outside of West Africa. The contrast between the death rates of the 4WIR and that of the white regiments stationed in Gibraltar at the same time was obvious: 'the mortality was at least four times as high'.[70] The explicit comparison between white and black mortality in a single clearly defined location, where other variables such as proximity to marshes, accommodation and diet were not a factor, was deemed to be proof that Europe was inhabitable only by white people and that black people could not thrive in a temperate climate. Gibraltar was far from being a cold locale, and indeed many from Britain or the northern states of America would have

[67] Review of Boudin's 'Statistics of the sanitary condition and mortality of forces by land and sea, as influenced by season, localities, age, race and national characters', *Edinburgh Medical and Surgical Journal* 67 (1847), 527.
[68] Nott and Gliddon, *Indigenous Races of the Earth*, 378, 398.
[69] *Littell's Living Age* 22 (1849), 175; 'Man's power of adaptation to different climates', *Pennsylvania Journal of Prison Discipline and Philanthropy* 5 (1850), 9; Philip C. Williams, 'On acclimation', *The Medical Examiner and Record of Medical Science* 68 (1850), 447.
[70] Alexander M. Tulloch, *Statistical Reports on the Sickness, Mortality and Invaliding among the Troops in the United Kingdom, the Mediterranean and British America* (London: HM Stationery Office, 1839), 18a.

found it uncomfortably hot for much of the year. But unlike the West Indies, or West Africa, Gibraltar had a noticeably cooler winter. And if the black troops of the 4WIR struggled in Gibraltar, then a posting to even colder climes could not be countenanced.

In fact, far more was made of the data from Gibraltar than was really merited. During the two years the 4WIR was stationed there, the regiment lost 119 of its members (12 per cent) to disease, mainly from lung complaints, but a mortality rate of 6 per cent per year, while higher than average for black regiments (3–4 per cent according to Tulloch's data between 1817 and 1836), was not untypical for the early nineteenth century. Between January 1808 and December 1812, for example, the 4WIR undertook garrison duty in Surinam (1808), Martinique (1809) and Guadeloupe (1810–12). The regiment reported an average of five deaths per month, or sixty deaths (6 per cent) a year, exactly the same rate as that experienced in Gibraltar.[71] The wider context of the Gibraltar data, which Tulloch had mentioned in his report as 'it very little exceeded the ratio to which the Negro is occasionally subject', was completely lost, or deliberately ignored, as publications reviewed or reprinted the information. The key point stressed again and again was that black troops who had enjoyed the same conditions as white troops, even sharing the same barracks, had died in greater numbers from lung complaints. The *American Journal of the Medical Sciences* thought the data clearly showed 'the unfitness of the constitution of the negro for any other than his native climate', and as for the *London Medical Gazette,* it highlighted 'a naturally greater predisposition to consumption in the negro'.[72] By 1848 the sufferings of the 4WIR in Gibraltar had morphed into a 'fearful mortality' in one publication, while British ethnologist James Hunt claimed the 4WIR had 'nearly all perished of pulmonary disease in fifteen months', proving that 'the farther they go north, the higher becomes the rate of mortality'. Hunt made this claim in an address to the Ethnological Society while Tulloch himself was in audience. Curiously, although Tulloch asked a question at the end, he did not attempt to correct Hunt's erroneous claims relating to the 4WIR in Gibraltar.[73] In fact, such claims were not based on any

---

71 Monthly returns of the 4WIR in WO27/251-253.
72 Tulloch, *Statistical Reports on the...United Kingdom*, 17a; *American Journal of the Medical Sciences*, 1 [1841], 450; 'Observations on the statistics of phthisis', *London Medical Gazette* N.S. 2 (1842), 828.
73 *Monthly Retrospect of the Medical Sciences* 1 (1848), 230; James Hunt, 'On ethnoclimatology; or the acclimatization of man', *Transactions of the Ethnological Society of London* 2 (1863), 75, 82. There is no evidence in the surviving records of the Ethnological Society that Tulloch was ever a member.

evidence whatsoever. When the 4WIR was disbanded in early 1819, and the former soldiers resettled in Sierra Leone, 950 men were on the transports to West Africa, including 860 rank-and-file soldiers.[74] Of course these War Office records were not widely accessible, even to those with the inclination to check, but Tulloch, who was the main source for these authors, had not claimed that the regiment had been devastated, merely that the mortality was higher than for the white regiments stationed alongside the 4WIR. The exaggeration of the mortality of the 4WIR was done deliberately to bolster the argument of Nott, and other polygenists, that each race of man had a defined space on earth, preordained by a creator perhaps, and to move beyond it was simply to invite higher death rates that would eventually lead to extinction.

Polygenism had many strings to its bow, and the WIRs, as the most heavily studied body of black men in the world, provided a vital source of corroborating evidence. Aside from the argument of unique adaptability to geographic-specific disease environments that was only possible if races were unchangingly different from each other, polygenists routinely exaggerated the significance of physical differences between races, particularly those claimed by Morton's measurements of skull capacities. Charles Hamilton Smith, who rose to the rank of lieutenant colonel in the British army before turning to natural history in his retirement, reported that when military caps were issued to new recruits of the 2WIR, 'it was observed, that scarcely any fitted the heads of the privates excepting the two smallest sizes; in many cases robust men, of the standard height, required padding an inch and a half in thickness, to fit their caps'.[75] Old arguments about the need to treat white and black patients differently also re-emerged with added energy and impetus. Mississippian Samuel Cartwright, who like many other Southern physicians had travelled to Europe and the West Indies, placed great faith in statistical medicine since it 'discloses truth, which often lies too deeply hid to be uncovered by the labor of any one individual practitioner of medicine'. He was also well aware of the valuable contribution made by 'the medical men attached to the Prussian, French and British armies and navies'.[76] In a number of

---

[74] Monthly return for Gibraltar February 1819, WO17/1805.

[75] Charles Hamilton Smith, *The Natural History of the Human Species* (Boston: Gould and Lincoln, 1851), 201. Smith's *Costumes of the Army of the British Empire* (London: Colnaghi and Co., 1812) contained one of the first published images of a WIR solider in uniform.

[76] Samuel Cartwright, 'Statistical medicine or numerical analysis applied to the investigation of morbid actions', *Western Journal of Medicine and Surgery* 1 (1848), 186, 195; Christopher D. E. Willoughby, 'Running away from drapetomania: Samuel A. Cartwright, medicine, and race in the antebellum South', *Journal of Southern History*, 84 (2018), 588–9.

articles on race and disease Cartwright cautioned that 'the same medical treatment which would benefit or cure a white man, would often injure or kill a negro, because of the differences in the organic or physical characters imprinted by the hand of nature on the two races'.[77] These differences were 'more deep, durable, and indelible' than just skin colour. Every part of the anatomy was 'tinctured with a shade of the pervading darkness'. Even the 'bones are whiter and harder than those of the white race, owing to their containing more phosphate of lime and less gelatine'. Moreover, unlike some army surgeons who believed the tougher skin of WIR soldiers prevented the use of bleeding as a treatment, Cartwright thought that black people were 'difficult to bleed, owing to the smallness of their veins'.[78] Maryland physician W. S. Forwood similarly cautioned his readers that as black patients could not 'bear depletion to the same extent', any attempt to use blood-letting would likely terminate fatally. Hereditary physical differences, he noted, meant black people 'cannot support the effects of active medicines with the same degree of impunity that is manifested by the white race'.[79]

Some went so far in their attempts to portray black people as physically inferior to whites that they contradicted previous publications relating to the WIRs and inadvertently challenged one of the main justifications for slavery. H. A. Ramsay argued that the 'Southern Negro physically and intellectually, [is] ... emphatically dissimilar to his bipedal fellow of the white race'. Although well-adapted to warmer climates, the black man 'cannot bear the same amount of physical endurance, or medical drasticity the white man can', due to the fact that his muscles were 'softer'.[80] This was indeed a remarkable claim, given that the perceived strength and endurance of black people in tropical conditions had underpinned the system of slavery for centuries. Edward Long had claimed back in 1774 that 'it is certain, that the Negroes, so far from suffering any inconveniences, are found to labour with most alacrity and ease to themselves in the very hottest part of the day'.[81] And, as discussed in Chapters 2 and 3, the ability of black soldiers to

---

[77] Samuel Cartwright, 'Report on the diseases and physical peculiarities of the negro race', *Southern Medical Reports* 2 (1850), 421. See also John S. Haller, 'The negro and the southern physician: a study of medical and racial attitudes, 1800–1860', *Medical History* 16 (1972), 238–53, especially 250.

[78] Dr Cartwright, 'Diseases and peculiarities of the negro race', *De Bow's Review* 9 (1851), 65, 69.

[79] W. S. Forwood, 'The negro – a distinct species', *Medical and Surgical Reporter* 10 (1857), 235.

[80] H. A. Ramsay, *The Necrological Appearances of Southern Typhoid Fever in the Negro* (Columbia: Constitutionalist Office, 1852), 13.

[81] Long, *History of Jamaica*, II, 412.

undergo fatiguing marches under the heat of a West Indian sun had been remarked on again and again by WIR commanders and by the medical personnel attached to the army.

None of these arguments went uncontested. Some writers simply deplored the blurring of the lines between politics and medicine: 'Make our medical journals politico-medical organs, and farewell to science! Farewell to truth!' Others stuck doggedly to the alternative interpretation that the different races were simple varieties and not different species, in much the same way that a terrier and a Labrador were both dogs. Most doctors had never 'indulged in the absurdity of attributing to the Negro different physiological laws from those which govern the Caucasian'.[82] After publishing a highly critical review of *Types of Mankind* in 1854, which castigated Nott and Gliddon for twisting facts 'to enable them to prove the negro to be of a different origin from the white man', the editors of the *Charleston Medical Journal* wished to set out clearly their own view: 'That all the races of men, including the negro, are of one species and of one origin. That the negro is a striking and now permanent variety, like the numerous varieties in domesticated animals'.[83] The same publication's review of *Indigenous Races* a few years later was even more scathing. The book presented 'nothing new, or worthy of notice' and had singularly failed to prove 'that there is any anatomical difference' between men, and, as far as the *Charleston Medical Journal* was concerned, 'science has not disproved the doctrine' of the Bible.[84] Even in a state like South Carolina, where slavery formed the backbone of the economy and the entire society was constructed around the subjugation of black people, there were plenty who thought Nott was fundamentally wrong.

A rare African voice speaking out against the polygenists belonged to James Africanus Beale Horton. Horton, a native of Sierra Leone, together with his compatriot William Broughton Davies, received his medical training at the University of Edinburgh, before being commissioned for West African service by the British army in 1859.[85] Although formally staff surgeons, and not attached to the WIRs based in Africa, the pair served throughout West Africa, including on campaigns against the Asante where WIR soldiers were present. As a literate and well-educated African, Horton was outraged at the deprecation

[82] *Charleston Medical Journal* 7 (1852), 92, 94.
[83] *Charleston Medical Journal* 9 (1854), 630, 657.
[84] *Charleston Medical journal* 12 (1857), 651–2.
[85] *Commissioned Officers in the Medical Service of the British Army, 1660–1960* (London: Wellcome Historical Medical Library, 1968), 425.

of his countrymen by armchair anthropologists who knew 'nothing of the negro race'. He did not deny that Africans were comparatively uncivilised compared to Europeans, but this was readily attributed to the 'damaging influences to which the negro race has for centuries been subjected'. Given the opportunity he was convinced that Africans could be the equal of Europeans. Horton reserved particular ire for the polygenists, whose work he considered to be 'so barefacedly false, so utterly the subversion of scientific truth' and based on ideas 'which only exist in their imagination'. On behalf of his fellow Africans, he claimed 'the existence of the attribute of a common humanity in the African or negro race; that there exist no radical distinctions between him and his more civilised *confrère*'.[86]

Most critics of polygenesis based their opposition on religious rather than medical or humanitarian grounds. Nott's airy dismissal of established and accepted biblical chronology rankled with many who used the works of naturalists such as Prichard to refute his polygenist ideas.[87] A few authors, however, dared to challenge Nott on his use of medical evidence. John Bachman ridiculed the oft-repeated claim that mulattoes were infertile, noting that the most recent United States census had reported more than 400,000 mulattoes and that the population was increasing.[88] Some challenged Nott directly, relating to comparative disease susceptibility and mortality. The anonymous reviewer of *Indigenous Races* for the *Southern Medical and Surgical Journal*, while not tackling the 'learned author' over his wider argument in favour of polygenesis, could not agree that 'negroes are comparatively exempt from all the endemic diseases of the south'. In fact, it was his experience that away from the rice coast, 'negroes suffer equally with the whites, annual attacks of intermittent and remittent fevers, dysentery, malarial pneumonia &c'. Supposing that the 'error' arose because 'negroes are comparatively exempt from fever upon the rice and cotton plantations of the low-country', the reality was that 'no length of residence, nor even nativity, affords the least immunity either to the white or to the black man'.[89] If, for this author, the flaw in Nott's argument was

---

[86] James Africanus B. Horton, *West African Countries and Peoples, British and Native* (London: John Churchill, 1868), 29, 35–7.

[87] See, for example, Abraham Coles, *A Critique on Nott and Gliddon's Ethnological Works* (Burlington: Medical and Surgical Reporter, 1857), and *Protestant Episcopal Quarterly Review* 1 (1858), 1–25. See also Christopher A. Luse, 'Slavery's champions stood at odds: polygenesis and the defense of slavery', *Civil War History* 53 (2007), 379–412, and Kidd, *Forging of Races*, 121–68.

[88] John Bachman, 'An examination of the characteristics of genera', *Charleston Medical Journal* 10 (1855), 208.

[89] *Southern Medical and Surgical Journal* 14 (1858), 22.

that neither whites nor blacks acquired immunity to inland fevers, for E. D. Fenner the flaw was that both races could evidently acquire immunity to the typical fevers of New Orleans. It was, he wrote, 'universally admitted that all immigrants from more northern regions to the south were very liable to suffer from the endemic fevers, for the first two or three years of their residence, but that after that period they obtain comparative health here as they did where they came from, and some of them much better'.[90] Thus two different medical authorities challenged Nott from opposite positions but with the same central point, that diseases affected whites and blacks in similar ways and that acclimation could be gained, or not, regardless of race.

Contemporary writers taking issue with Nott's medical arguments were far outnumbered by those who challenged him on religious grounds. The same has proved true of historians.[91] The key difference between the medical case for polygenesis and other arguments in support of it was that Nott was able to draw on first the publications of army surgeons, such as Moseley, Hunter, Jackson and Fergusson who had already clearly established that black bodies, particularly those belonging to the men of the WIRs, were fundamentally divergent from white ones, and capable of different things. And second, Nott could cite a set of supposedly unbiased and official medical statistics gathered by the British army and published by the British Parliament. They seemed to have official sanction and approval, and constituted hard data, not supposition or interpretation, and thus were difficult to challenge without alternative sources. Unless Tulloch's work was completely fabricated, and no one claimed it was, then without doubt it provided a whole host of supporting evidence to those who promoted the idea that unalterable and everlasting differences between the races actually existed. While it would be going too far to suggest that the writings of WIR surgeons about black bodies led directly to the emergence of ethnology as a science, or of polygenesis as a popular theory, it is evident that these publications were of immense importance. As this chapter has demonstrated, the unique perspectives offered by those who had worked alongside the men of the WIRs ultimately underpinned several key polygenist arguments relating to the origins of humanity.

---

[90] E. D. Fenner, 'Acclimation; and the liability of negroes to the endemic fevers of the south', *Southern Medical and Surgical Journal* 14 (1858), 454.

[91] See, for example, Terence D. Keel, 'Religion, polygenism and the early science of human origins', *History of the Human Sciences* 26 (2013), 3–32.

6   Damage Done: The Asante Campaigns

In November 1859 Charles Darwin published his long-awaited *On the Origin of Species*. Drawing on the data collected during his extensive voyages on the *Beagle* between 1831 and 1836, Darwin demonstrated how evolution by natural selection occurred. Others had argued that species could change over long periods of time as they adapted to their environments, but Darwin was the first to explain clearly why it happened. Individuals who adapted best were most likely to survive and breed, and thus, over many generations, beneficial traits would be passed on. Species that had started out as united would diverge as their specific environments altered. Darwin wrote about animals, not humans, but the consequences for those who had debated the origins of humanity for the previous century were obvious for all to see. Humanity, after all, was simply a uniquely clever form of animal, and Darwin's logic was inescapable: humans must have evolved, along with other primates, from a common ape ancestor. But Darwin had not only undermined those who believed that differences between Europeans, Asians and Africans were immutable, and that polygenesis was the only explanation for these differences, he had dismantled the idea of any kind of 'genesis' at all. Natural selection was brutal, random at times, and left little room for God.[1]

Darwin's work circulated rapidly, particularly among anglophone intellectuals. In the United States the most strident of the polygenists, Josiah Nott, thought Darwin was 'clearly crazy', though his effective demolition of biblical chronology was 'a capital dig into the parsons'.[2] Nott's world was, of course, about to be turned upside down. Within months of him writing this, most of the southern states had left the United States, and by April 1861 war had broken out. Few Americans had the time or inclination to engage in debates about the origins of

---

[1] Cynthia Eagle Russett, *Darwin in America: the Intellectual Response, 1865–1912* (San Francisco: W. H. Freeman, 1976), 3, 31; B. Riccardo Brown, *Until Darwin, Science, Human Variety and the Origins of Race* (London: Pickering and Chatto, 2010), 99.
[2] Nott to Squier, 22 August 1860, E. G. Squier Papers, Library of Congress.

humanity during a period of national, regional and personal crisis, but after the war ended in 1865 ethnological discussions gradually resumed. With slavery abolished, one of the crucial antebellum underpinnings of the polygenesis argument – the need to justify the enslavement of an entire race – had gone, but it was readily replaced by a new need to delineate clearly the key differences between white and black people. The meaning of emancipation was hotly contested. Freedpeople, and some Radical Republicans, hoped it meant equality. White southerners were adamant that it meant nothing of the sort, and a great deal of intellectual energy would be expended over the coming decades to reestablish white superiority.[3] Some of the energy came from Josiah Nott.

Although a sympathetic retrospective published in the early twentieth century claimed that Nott came 'to accept to the full all of Darwin's views and conclusions', the evidence from his contemporary writings is much more ambivalent.[4] Nott acknowledged and did not attempt to dismantle what he termed 'development theory', but he did seek to marginalise it by pointing out that it required hundreds of thousands, if not millions, of years to test empirically. As far as human societies were concerned, Darwin was irrelevant since 'during the lifetime of a nation' (measured in centuries rather than millennia) blacks could not transform into whites or vice versa. Nott did not believe the new development theory had actually provided a 'conclusive argument in proof of the unity of the human family', but there was a significant shift in emphasis in his argument after the Civil War. Polygenesis *per se* was barely mentioned; instead the role of blood in transferring permanent traits between generations became the focus. Claiming that impure blood 'cannot be washed out in many generations', Nott promoted the idea of hereditary 'instincts' that included intellect, abilities in the arts and sciences, and agricultural innovation. Inevitably, he thought that newly freed slaves could not attain the heights of civilisation achieved by the white man since they would be held back by a 'small brain, inferior intellect, and instinctive dislike to agricultural labor'.[5] Writing to the superintendent of the Freedmen's Bureau in 1866, Nott went so far as to claim that former slaves were 'doomed to extermination' now that whites were no longer obliged to care and provide for them. There was nothing that anyone could do to close the gap between white and black

---

[3] Two of the best summaries of Reconstruction are Eric Foner, *Reconstruction: America's Unfinished Revolution, 1863–1877* (New York: Harper and Row, 1988), and John Hope Franklin, *Reconstruction after the Civil War* (Chicago: University of Chicago Press, 1961).

[4] William M. Polk, 'Josiah C. Nott', *American Journal of Obstetrics* 67 (1913), 957.

[5] J. C. Nott, *Instincts of Races* (New Orleans: L. Graham, 1866), 3, 5, 28.

people since 'the diversity of races as it exists can only be regarded as the work of the Almighty'. There is irony in the fact that Nott cloaked his racism in religion, given his disdain for theology throughout his career.[6]

As Nott gradually abandoned polygenism, an argument that by the mid 1860s seemed to have had its day, he found succour for his racism in a somewhat unlikely place. Charles Darwin had read Nott's work on polygenesis, and although he did not agree with it, as early as 1859 he had commented privately that the struggle between races would lead to 'the less intellectual races being exterminated'.[7] Of course, Darwin was not the first to suggest that the future demographic prospects for Africans were gloomy. Alexander Tulloch had said the same thing in the 1830s, and polygenists such as Nott and Robert Knox had welcomed what one historian terms the 'extinction discourse' long before Darwin chimed in.[8] But by the time Darwin published *The Descent of Man* in 1871, he thought it was self-evident that the white race had proved its superiority over the other races many times, and the inevitable outcome of history would be an 'evolutionary war' that would result in the extinction of non-white races. Only the 'fittest' would survive.[9] As Douglas Lorimer has noted, this fitted neatly with the popular Victorian idea of the 'great chain of being' that placed white people at the pinnacle of the races and black people at the very bottom.[10] Thus even Charles Darwin, an intellectual giant whose personal humanitarianism is well established, could not avoid unthinkingly following popular conceptions of so-called higher and lower races when discussing the struggle for life. For racists like Nott, intent on putting freedpeople firmly back under white control, the acceptance that there were superior and inferior races was a crucial concession, and Nott made efforts to establish that white supremacy was simply a case of restoring what he considered to be the natural order of things.

Absent from Nott's post-war writings is any discussion of the medical differences between whites and blacks that had been so central to

---

[6] J. C. Nott, 'The negro race', *Popular Magazine of Anthropology* 1 (1866), 115–16.

[7] John C. Greene, 'Darwin as a social evolutionist', *Journal of the History of Biology* 10 (1977), 4, 6.

[8] Patrick Brantlinger, *Dark Vanishings: Discourse on the Extinction of Primitive Races, 1800–1930* (Ithaca: Cornell University Press, 2003), 1, 44, 164–6.

[9] Charles Darwin, *The Descent of Man and Selection in Relation to Sex* (London: John Murray, 1871); Edward Beasley, *The Victorian Reinvention of Race* (London: Routledge, 2010), 100; Evelleen Richards, 'The "moral anatomy" of Robert Knox: the interplay between biological and social thought in Victorian scientific naturalism', *Journal of the History of Biology* 22 (1989), 434; Edward Beasley, 'Making races', *Victorian Review* 40 (2014), 50.

[10] Douglas A. Lorimer, *Colour, Class and the Victorians: English Attitudes to the Negro in the Mid-Nineteenth Century* (Leicester: Leicester University Press, 1978), 133.

his antebellum polygenist thesis. He evidently thought that his new racist theories based on blood and heredity had more potency in the era of emancipation. Others did not relinquish ideas relating to the intersection of race and medicine quite so readily, and the lingering influence of Tulloch and others who had written on the subject is readily apparent in the writings of WIR surgeons in the second half of the nineteenth century. Lasting damage to the medical reputation of black soldiers had been done. No longer would surgeons praise the special superhuman abilities afforded to WIR soldiers by black skin, eyes and ears. Instead, medical weaknesses now featured prominently. Although far from being the first to highlight the unusual vulnerability of black soldiers to lung complaints, phthisis in particular, Tulloch had brought it to the attention of a wide audience. Medical and ethnological writers of the 1840s and 1850s, as Chapter 5 outlined, continuously referenced the experiences of the 4WIR in Gibraltar as proof of 'some inherent weakness of constitution in the negro which renders him peculiarly liable to phthisis'. By the 1860s regimental surgeons serving with the WIRs fully accepted that high numbers of phthisis cases among their soldiers were 'owing to constitutional predisposition', that soldiers were 'naturally predisposed' to the disease and even that it was 'hereditary'.[11] Some thought that certain environmental circumstances exacerbated this innate vulnerability. James Barry, staff surgeon in the Bahamas in 1870, blamed 'improper clothing, bad diet, excessive venery, a habit of covering up the face and their inhaling air loaded with foetid exhalations from the negro skin'.[12] Others blamed the weather, especially when there had been 'cold northerly winds and the heavy dews at night' or 'exposure to a draught whilst the body was perspiring'.[13] In 1867 the surgeon attached to the 4WIR attributed the prevalence of consumption among black soldiers to 'the venereal poison acting on a constitution weakened by sexual excess commenced at a very early age'.[14]

Most commonly, though, the high number of lung complaints was attributed to a simple, inherent and universal fault with black male bodies. Andrew Robertson Smith, staff surgeon at Up Park Camp in Jamaica,

---

[11] Report for Sierra Leone, 1870, WO334/155; Sanitary reports for Belize, Jamaica and Trinidad, 1861, WO334/132. Philip Curtin points out that tuberculosis was comparatively rare in Africa and that the disease takes a long period to establish itself in a community. Mortality among black troops, he notes, peaked in the 1870s in the West Indies and the 1880s in West Africa. Philip D. Curtin, 'African health at home and abroad', *Social Science History* 10 (1986), 381–3.

[12] Sanitary report for the Bahamas, 1870, WO334/161.

[13] Sanitary report for the Bahamas, 1861, WO334/132; Sanitary report for Jamaica, 1869, WO334/155.

[14] *Army Medical Department Report for the Year 1867* (London: HMSO, 1869), 72.

complained that 'many of the men have badly formed chests' and that 'their chest capacity on an average is inferior to the European soldier'.[15] Such was the new fixation on lung capacity, and the belief that a smaller than average capacity indicated someone prone to pulmonary diseases, that undersized chest measurement was the single most frequent reason given for rejecting new recruits into the WIRs.[16] This argument had never been made before Tulloch's publications of the late 1830s and early 1840s. In fact, data on chest measurements and supposed lung capacity, unlike that for height, was simply not collected. But by the 1860s and 1870s military surgeons attached to the WIRs had been absorbing the work of Tulloch and those who followed him in writing about differential racial vulnerability to disease, for more than twenty years. Andrew Robertson Smith, for example, had joined the army medical staff only in 1856.[17] By then the medical vulnerability of black people generally, and WIR soldiers in particular, had become a well-established fact of medical and statistical literature. It was their black bodies that made WIR soldiers vulnerable, and few thought to investigate further.

The reports submitted by regimental surgeons were internal army documents, but in 1859 the British government began publishing annual *Statistical, Sanitary and Medical Reports* that included a lengthy section on troop mortality throughout the British Empire. The published volumes used edited versions of the annual reports from regimental surgeons and brought them to the attention of a much broader audience. Clearly modelled on the pioneering work of Tulloch in the 1830s and 1840s, these statistics continued to erode much older orthodoxies about the health advantages enjoyed by WIR troops in tropical climates. While offering a great deal of medical detail, the most significant statistics for white and black troops stationed in the West Indies compared the proportion of hospital admissions, the mortality rate and the time needed for recuperation. In virtually every year between 1859 and 1900 the data for white troops was better than for black troops. In Jamaica in 1864, for example, hospital admissions were 30 per cent higher for black troops, the average length of a hospital stay was nine days longer and the overall mortality rate was no less than five times higher.[18] In 1876 hospital admissions were 58 per cent higher for

[15]   Sanitary reports for Jamaica, 1869 and 1870, WO334/155, WO334/161.

[16]   *Army Medical Department Report for the Year 1897* (London: HMSO, 1899), 116; *Army Medical Department Report for the Year 1900* (London: HMSO, 1902), 103, 111.

[17]   A. Peterkin and William Johnston, *Commissioned Officers in the Medical Service of the British Army, 1660–1960* (London: Wellcome Library, 1968), I, 387.

[18]   *Statistical, Sanitary and Medical Reports for 1862* (London: HMSO, 1864), 70, 74, 79.

black troops, the proportion reporting sick at any one time was 34 per cent higher and the mortality rate was six times higher.[19] The data for black troops only improved marginally as the century drew to a close. In 1898 hospital admissions were 76 per cent higher for black troops, the proportion reporting sick at any one time was 15 per cent higher and the mortality rate remained double that for white troops. These figures were almost the exact inverse of what had been the norm for the early decades of the nineteenth century.

The figures really only told one story: that white military mortality and sickness rates in the Caribbean were much better in the latter half of the nineteenth century than they had been in eighteenth and early nineteenth centuries. In part this was because there were far fewer white soldiers in the West Indies, reflecting its marginal imperial position in the later nineteenth century. The island possessions faced no meaningful external threat, and their economic worth to the empire had waned as India's had waxed. In 1796 there had been more than 20,000 British troops on active service in the Caribbean, and even the peacetime strength of the white regiments between 1817 and 1836 averaged 4,333.[20] By 1890 there were just 1,044 British soldiers in the region, the vast majority of whom were stationed either in Barbados (long regarded at the healthiest island for white troops) or at Newcastle in Jamaica, at an elevation of 4,000 feet, where disease-spreading mosquitoes were rarely to be found.[21] But other changes implemented following Tulloch's report in 1838 had clearly had an impact. White troops now served in the West Indies for a shorter period and enjoyed better quality food and accommodation than their predecessors.

The same cannot be said for the WIRs, where mortality and sickness rates only declined marginally when compared to the early nineteenth century. Surgeons compiling the reports had various explanations for the figures. Some pointed to the fact that, unlike white troops, the WIR soldiers did not receive a compulsory supper and instead were expected to fend for themselves for an evening meal. Others blamed the fact that 'the black soldiers seldom wear their boots or shoes except when on duty' that left them vulnerable to foot injuries, or that excessive 'night duties' that exposed them to cold night air.[22] As we saw in Chapter 3, racist ideas that black people required less sleep than white people meant WIR soldiers were assigned night duties at twice the rate of white soldiers.

---

[19] *Army Medical Department Report for the Year 1876* (London: HMSO, 1877), 89, 92.

[20] British Library, Stowe MSS 921; *Statistical Report for the West Indies*, 5.

[21] *Army Medical Report 1890* (London: HMSO, 1892), 83.

[22] Sanitary reports for Jamaica, Belize and St Lucia, 1861, WO334/132; Sanitary report for Jamaica, 1869, WO334/155.

This was still the case in the 1860s, with the regimental surgeon in Georgetown, Guyana, admitting that the men of the 1WIR had 'too few nights in bed'.[23] The men themselves were apportioned some of the blame for high sickness rates, both for being 'so abominably filthy in habits and so indolent that they often empty their slops immediately outside the wooden huts' enabling infections to spread easily, but also, as Andrew Robertson Smith in Jamaica complained, because 'they are particularly fond of concealing their diseases and trying to treat themselves'.[24] Nothing was probably more frustrating for a surgeon, fresh from Edinburgh's medical school, to find the men using folk medicine instead of seeking his counsel. The particular recruitment and rotation practices of the WIRs also took its toll. In 1864 Dr Bent, the principal medical officer in Jamaica, blamed the excessive sickness and mortality among black troops on the island on the 5WIR 'being throughout the year in course of formation, and consisting of recruits, chiefly miserable boys, half starved and half grown'. The fact that the 4WIR had left behind 'the more sickly men' when it embarked for Africa, and the recently returned 1WIR had numerous men suffering 'the effects of previous African service', clearly had not helped. Higher than average rates of medical discharge in 1864 were attributed to 'the exposure and privations of the men engaged in the Ashantee campaign'.[25] As well as several protracted campaigns against the Asante, the WIRs were deployed against a variety of smaller African states at odds with the expansionist British. Deaths in battle, or from wounds received, occurred regularly, and temporary army camps were periodically swept by dysentery. High rates of sickness could readily be attributed to 'fatigue and exposure incident to a march of 150 miles in the African bush' as each night the men erected huts made 'of a bamboo framework, roofed with palm and banana leaves' that provided little 'proper shelter from the heavy rains'.[26] Above all, however, the excessive vulnerability of black troops to 'tubercular diseases' was cited time and again as a reason for high rates of mortality.[27] Few physicians attempted to establish anything other than a simple racial explanation for the data.

[23] *Statistical, Sanitary and Medical Reports for 1861* (London: HMSO, 1863), 264.
[24] Sanitary reports for the Bahamas and Jamaica, 1870, WO334/161.
[25] *Statistical, Sanitary and Medical Reports for 1862* (London: HMSO, 1864), 74, 78.
[26] *Army Medical Department Report for the year 1896* (London: HMSO, 1898), 104; J. E. Caulfeild, *One Hundred Years' History of the 2nd Batt: West India Regiment* (London: Forster Groom, 1899), 150. See also J. A. B. Horton, *The Diseases of Tropical Climates and Their Treatment* (London: J. and A. Churchill, 1874), 228.
[27] The post-mortem dissections of those who succumbed to other illness also regularly found 'tubercular deposits … in the lungs'. *Statistical, Sanitary and Medical Reports for 1864* (London: HMSO, 1866), 69.

Given the disparity in sickness and mortality rates of white and black soldiers in the West Indies, one might ask why there was no attempt to dispense with the services of the WIRs altogether and make do with white regiments. The answer lies in a continued acceptance that certain Caribbean locations remained too deadly for white troops. Fort Augusta in Kingston harbour or Prince Rupert's Head in Dominica, labelled 'the Golgotha of the Antilles' by one WIR officer, had not suddenly become healthy overnight.[28] The *Naval and Military Gazette* enthusiastically supported the re-creation of 4WIR in 1862 thinking the army 'could most usefully employ them where service is deadly to white troops', a sentiment that would not have been out of place half a century earlier. The same publication a year later somewhat exaggeratedly claimed that 'the West Indies will always be the English Algeria'.[29] By the 1860s this was clearly no longer true as white regiments were perfectly able to withstand a posting to the West Indies, but the WIRs clearly remained useful, despite their comparatively high sickness and mortality rates, because they helped to preserve British lives, just as they had done since 1795.

The mortality data for WIR troops serving in West Africa was little better than for their counterparts in the Caribbean. Tulloch's 1840 volume on West Africa had suggested that WIR troops enjoyed the best health on service in their 'native climate', but the data from the second half of the nineteenth century suggested something rather different. In a good year hospitalisation rates were only 140 per cent and death rates 1.5 per cent; in a bad year they were double that. Since 1830, when the last white troops had been removed from British colonies in West Africa, both garrison and offensive duties had been undertaken by black troops. The decision had been justified as saving the lives of European soldiers and an 'immediate decrease took place' in both hospital admissions and mortality rates in the African colonies. Before 1830 hospitalisation rates of white troops had been as high as 297 per cent with mortality rates of 48 per cent. Such figures were unsustainable, a force dispatched from Britain would be almost completely wiped out within two years. Comparable rates for the WIRs in the year they assumed sole responsibility for West African operations were 72 per cent and 1.6 per cent, respectively.[30]

---

[28] Luke Smyth O'Connor, 'Twelve months service in western Africa', *United Service Journal* (1846), pt 1, 222.

[29] *Naval and Military Gazette*, 15 February 1862 and 15 August 1863.

[30] Surgeon-Major Albert A. Gore, *A Contribution to the Medical History of Our West African Campaign* (London: Bailliere, Tindall and Cox, 1876), 208. See also John Rankin, *Healing the African Body: British Medicine in West Africa, 1800–1860* (Columbia: University of Missouri Press, 2015), 135.

When these figures were set alongside the data for white troops, the posting of the WIRs to West Africa was fully justified from a medical standpoint. After 1830, however, there were no really comparable statistics since the only white troops in West Africa were WIR officers and a few Royal Artillery personnel. Thus, the comparison most often made was between data for West Africa and that for the West Indies, where white mortality had fallen dramatically since the early years of the nineteenth century. More often than not, data for the WIR troops serving in West Africa was worse than for counterparts in the West Indies. In 1889, for example, WIR soldiers serving in West Africa were twice as likely as those in the Caribbean to spend time in hospital, and the mortality rate was 69 per cent higher. In 1894 the mortality rate was twice as high in Africa.[31]

There was a significant and permanent shift in attitudes towards black troops in general and the WIRs in particular during the 1860s and 1870s. The change was prompted and accelerated by two campaigns against the Asante people in modern-day Ghana, the first in 1864 and the second in 1873–4. The staff assistant surgeon on the Gold Coast in 1864 was William Alexander Gardiner. His report on the Asante campaign of that year was published in full, as well as being reprinted in the press, and the WIRs were not depicted positively. While accepting that the 4WIR had endured 'constant fatigue duties', including constructing new buildings for hospitals during persistent heavy rain, they had also 'suffered very considerably from dysentery and fevers of the intermittent and remittent classes'.[32] Even worse, reinforcements from the 1WIR 'suffered mostly from fever on their arrival'. What frustrated Gardiner was the fact that 'all West Indian soldiers suffer greatly from change of climate' should have been well known in London. Indeed they 'suffered more from the effects of this climate on their first arrival than white men would'.[33] This is an example of the influence that Tulloch's debunking of seasoning had on medical thought. A parliamentary report into an African expedition in 1841–2, written roughly contemporaneously to Tulloch's volume on Africa, stated 'that the constitution of the negro, whether of African or American birth, requires an habitual residence in Africa to be exempt from the fever of the country'. Seasoning was still believed possible in the early 1840s. By the 1860s it was 'not new

[31] *Army Medical Department Report for the Year 1889* (London: HMSO, 1891), 89, 94; *Army Medical Department Report for the Year 1894* (London: HMSO, 1896), 73, 77.

[32] *Statistical, Sanitary and Medical Reports for 1863* (London: HMSO, 1865), 329, 333. Gardiner's report on the 1864 campaign was included in the 1863 issue published in 1865 and reprinted in the *Naval and Military Gazette,* 4 November 1865.

[33] Ibid., 334–5.

information', as Gardiner rather testily pointed out, that West Indian soldiers would suffer from illnesses in Africa simply because they were not native to Africa.[34] They, like white soldiers, could never become fully adapted to the West African environment. Gardiner's opinion of black troops was probably also shaped by his experience of the medically unfit recruits he was sent. The 4WIR had been newly raised in the West Indies before being sent straight to Africa and consisted, he thought, of 'weakly men' and the cast-off 'weeds' of other regiments. Once in Africa the WIR soldier displayed 'none of the hardihood and spirited endurance of the white man', and when admitted to hospital 'he gives up all hope' and spent his time preparing for the end. This 'apathetic indifference to the future is inborn in the African character', Gardiner opined, and had infected 'their consanguineous brethren of the West Indies'.[35]

Andrew Clarke's internal army report to the secretary at war in 1864 on British possessions in West Africa confirmed and reinforced much of what Gardiner said. Clarke commanded the Royal Engineers on the Gold Coast between 1863 and 1864 and, while accepting that 'the climate is very unfavourable to European constitutions', he reported that the WIRs 'suffer almost as much, if not more, when taken to Western Africa, than would white men'. He accepted that some of this suffering could be attributed to the 'poor provision' made for the WIRs, since they often had to make do with 'mud huts, dark, ill-ventilated, and with no floors but the bare ground'. These were, he considered, of 'worse construction than the average of African hovels'. The army also struggled to find medical personnel willing to accept positions in West Africa.[36] Changes could be made to alleviate some of this distress of course, but nothing could be done about what he considered to be flaws in the intrinsic physicality of black West Indian bodies. Clarke made an important distinction between liberated Africans, whom he described as 'a fine body of men, clean, and soldier-like', and those recruited in the West Indies who 'do not form so good material for soldiers as the native Africans'. Gardiner had made a similar exception, amidst his general disdain for black troops, for the Gold Coast Corps. These African-born soldiers were 'fine, strong, hardy men, who bore the climate and exposure to the bush well'.[37] West Indians, by contrast,

[34] Ibid., 335–6.
[35] Ibid., 337.
[36] Memorandum on British possessions, west coast of Africa (1864), 21, 28, 53, 63–5, 101, WO33/13. For a biography of Clarke, see R. H. Vetch, *Life of Lieutenant-General the Hon. Sir Andrew Clarke* (London: J. Murray, 1905).
[37] *Statistical, Sanitary and Medical Reports for 1863* (London: HMSO, 1865), 336.

'suffered much from climate', and, more significantly, Clarke believed 'their powers of endurance, or of extra exertion, altogether fail when continuous exercise is called for'. This, of course, ran contrary to every account of the legendary stamina of the WIRs in the early decades of the nineteenth century. As Chapters 2 and 3 established, before 1840 superhuman abilities were attributed to all black WIR soldiers, even though they had been recruited from West Africa, East Africa, India, North America and the Caribbean. Black skin alone was deemed sufficient to provide protection against tropical illnesses. After 1860 these abilities were only attributed to West Africans. But while the native African recruits often displayed courage, Clarke believed that they 'are not so feared by their own race as are the white men', allowing him to claim that 'two-hundred white soldiers would be more than equal to the work that could be expected from the present number of about fifteen-hundred West Indian men'. Clarke's voice was clearly influential. His report was commissioned and then printed by the War Office for internal circulation among army commanders. While lauding the 'discipline, and admirable order of the West India Regiments', they were, he thought, on medical grounds no longer fit for purpose in West Africa.[38]

Clarke and Gardiner were part of a growing chorus of voices reporting on the physical and mental frailties of WIR soldiers. Samuel Rowe, assistant surgeon in the new colony of Lagos in 1869, retained a lingering faith in the efficacy of seasoning, observing 'the negro from the West Indies...goes through a process of acclimatisation to the malaria of the place as distinctly as does the European'. However, Rowe saw only a minor positive to the seasoning process as he thought it seemed to weaken the WIR soldier's 'vital power'. As a consequence of it 'his powers of resistance to and recovery from acute disease [such] as dysentery seem lessened' and it seemed clear that he would never match the health of locals.[39] The chief medical officer on the Gold Coast agreed that black soldiers had a 'low degree of vitality', when compared with European troops, while the governor of Lagos confessed that he lacked 'that confidence in the valour of the West India Regiments which they ought to inspire'.[40] Reports such as these, circulating among the higher echelons of Whitehall and the army, confirmed that the notion

---

[38] Memorandum on British possessions, west coast of Africa (1864), 65–6, WO33/13.

[39] Medical report Lagos, 1869, WO334/155. On Rowe's imperial career, see Spencer H. Brown, 'Colonialism on the cheap: a tale of two English army surgeons in Lagos, Samuel Rowe and Frank Simpson, 1862–1882', *The International Journal of African Historical Studies* 27 (1994), 551–88.

[40] Letter from Lagos, 20 April 1863; Memorandum on British possessions, west coast of Africa (1864), WO33/13, 59, 66, 100. Gold Coast report, 1868, WO334/36.

of the superhuman black soldier, prevalent in the early decades of the nineteenth century, was dead. Moreover, some of the army's annual medical reports were taken up by the press and given an even wider circulation. Under the headline 'Our Black Troops', the London *Times* reprinted the observations of Richard O'Flaherty, the senior medical officer in Jamaica, that 'the black soldier to outward view is apparently strong and muscular, but when sick, he has comparatively little power of resisting or sustaining disease'. This racial weakness, combined with 'continued exertion' and 'much heavier duty', explained why mortality in the WIRs in Jamaica was nearly three times that of white troops.[41] The original published report might have been perused by War Office officials, or senior staff at the Army Medical Department, and gone no further. The article in the *Times* was not only read by far more people, it was itself then reprinted in several British and American periodicals, awarding the information it contained the status of unquestioned truth. Indeed the *New York Medical Journal*, utilising comparable information from the Union army then operating in the Southern states, confirmed that 'the negro has not the ability to resist morbific influences which is possessed by the European, unless it is in the single matter of malarious diseases, and even in this, there is room for doubt'.[42]

This renewed assault on the medical fitness of black soldiers in the British army coincided with US army physicians discovering the black body for the first time. Some historians have suggested that those writing about the thousands of black soldiers serving with the Union army actually played an important part in shaping post-war attitudes towards black people more generally in the United States.[43] Sanford Hunt, a surgeon attached to the United States Volunteers, for instance reported that the black soldier 'fails to endure prolonged fatigue as well as the white man', that his supposed immunity to malaria 'has not been sustained by experience', and his 'tropical, or smaller, lung' left him uniquely vulnerable to pulmonary infections.[44] But it is crucially

---

[41] *Times* (UK), 19 September 1864. O'Flaherty's original report appeared in *Statistical, Sanitary and Medical Reports for 1862* (London: HMSO, 1864), 252–3.

[42] *New York Medical Journal* 1 (1865), 86; the original article was reprinted in the *British Medical Journal* 2 (1864), 497; *Army and Navy Gazette* 2 (1865), 250; *The Medical and Surgical Reporter* 12 (1865), 531; *Medical News and Library* 23 (1865), 15. Christine Bolt suggests that reports of the Morant Bay rebellion helped define Victorian attitudes towards West Indians, overlooking the numerous and largely negative reports circulating about the WIRs the year before. Christine Bolt, *Victorian Attitudes towards Race* (London: Routledge, 1971), 76.

[43] John S. Haller, *Outcasts from Evolution: Scientific Attitudes of Racial Inferiority, 1859–1900* (Chicago: University of Illinois Press, 1971), 21–34.

[44] Sanford B. Hunt, 'The negro as a solider', *Quarterly Journal of Psychological Medicine* 1 (1867), 166, 169, 175.

important to recall that contemporary writers investigating black soldiers in the United States were not starting from scratch. A significant
body of military-medical statistical literature already existed, indeed
some of it stretched back nearly thirty years and had reached very similar conclusions. And while we cannot be sure that Sanford Hunt had
read Tulloch and others who had written about the WIRs, he did cite
the work of Josiah Nott who, as Chapter 5 demonstrated, relied extensively on British military surgeons in his own publications.

Contemporary with the denial of the suitability of the WIR soldier for
African service was an attempt to rehabilitate the white soldier. Those
who pointed to the unfortunate fate of the Royal African Corps in the
1820s as an example of what happened to white soldiers in Africa were
placing far too much attention, some said, on an 'extremely dissipated,
unmanageable, and insubordinate' body of men. According to Albert
Gore, writing in Sierra Leone in 1867, poor accommodation, intem-
perance and general dissipated living all contributed towards excessive
white mortality in Africa and thus, he argued, 'it is really difficult to
say how far climatic influences act *per se* on the European constitution'
based solely on the evidence of medical statistics that were now nearly
forty years out of date.[45]

By the time Major General Garnet Wolseley took command of the
Asante campaign in 1873, the general perception of the military usefulness of WIR soldiers had declined significantly under a sustained
public and private assault. Wolseley, based on his reading of Clarke's
1864 report, and no doubt influenced by Gore who accompanied him
on the Asante campaign, considered that the WIRs 'are not physically
by any means as capable of withstanding the climate, still less exertion
and fatigue. It is a well-known fact here that Europeans suffer from the
climate less than black men from other localities'.[46] Given the information available to him, and his own deeply racist attitudes towards non-
whites, Wolseley immediately requested 'some of her Majesty's English
troops' be dispatched to West Africa for offensive operations.

Many in London believed that sending any white troops to Africa
was a recipe for disaster. The *Times*, for instance, reported on the fate
of nineteen white officers attached to the WIR at Cape Coast Castle.
Within a month 'only three had the strength to crawl about'. It cautioned against sending white regiments against the Asante in 1873 since

---

[45] *Army Medical Department Report for the Year 1867* (London: HMSO, 1869) 407, 415.
[46] Maj. Gen. Sir G. Wolseley to Edward Cardwell, Gold Coast forces, 13 October
1873, in Henry Brackenbury, *The Ashanti War: a Narration Prepared from the Official
Documents* (Edinburgh: William Blackwood, 1874), I, 191–2.

'they are sure to suffer very severely from sickness, as their comrades who have preceded them have already done, and a loss of life painful to contemplate will probably occur'.[47] Aware that there might be alarm in London at the thought of sending white troops to West Africa, Wolseley promised that all due medical precautions would be put in place, with pre-built hospitals and ships placed on standby to evacuate the sick and wounded, and that the soldiers would be used for no more than two months. Previous bad experiences, he assured them, had 'produced an exaggerated alarm as to the general influence of this climate upon European health'.[48] Wolseley was acutely aware of the importance of publicity and the press to the success of his campaign, and even before the war began he and his staff agreed that the 'apprehensions in the public mind' about African service needed to be addressed.[49] Deputy Surgeon General Anthony Home, like Gore before him, knew that the 'appalling loss' suffered by the Royal African Corps in the 1820s, together with the sustained mortality among WIR troops, meant that there was a need to revise 'a general opinion' against sending white troops to Africa. Authorities in London were therefore reminded that the Royal African Corps had been 'reckless, hopeless men' doing 'desperate service', lacking a good diet or proper housing.[50] The Asante campaign, with Britain's finest soldiers, would be different.

The campaign against the Asante fell naturally into two halves. The first, expelling an Asante incursion into the Gold Coast, took place mainly in November 1873 'without the assistance of any English troops'. A body of Royal Marines had disembarked in June 1873, but within a month most of them had come down with a fever, and by the end of July two-thirds were classed as 'ineffective' and the entire body was evacuated. This was hardly a good advert for the use of white troops in West Africa, but Anthony Home was quick to point out that the WIRs 'were almost as much foreigners on the Gold Coast as white men' and that they fell sick at nearly the same rate. The only difference was that the 'attacks of remittent fever in them were much milder than those seen in white men'.[51] Despite being 'very sickly', the men of 2WIR were not evacuated to Ascension Island like the marines but remained in Africa

[47] *Times,* 20 May 1864; 2 September 1873.
[48] Brackenbury, *The Ashanti War,* I, 192, 195.
[49] Ian F. W. Beckett, 'Manipulating the modern curse of armies: Wolseley, the press, and the Ashanti war, 1873–1874', in Stephen M. Miller (ed.), *Soldiers and Settlers in Africa, 1850–1918* (Brill: Leiden, 2009), 221–34.
[50] *Army Medical Department Report for the Year 1873* (London: HMSO, 1875), 236–7.
[51] Ibid., 218, 225, 238.

gradually recuperating. The WIRs, together with a sizeable force of local levies, eventually pushed the Asante out of the Gold Coast, but their success did not alter Home's opinion that white troops were 'absolutely essential' to the punitive expedition that Wolseley had planned against the Asante. Wolseley himself singled out numerous white officers for their 'hard work' in trying conditions during this first phase but made no mention whatsoever of the black troops who made up the bulk of his force. Indeed, in a letter to London he commented that 'however excellent' the officers of the WIRs were, the men 'must, from the very nature of their materials, be inferior'.[52]

Wolseley evidently had considerable influence in Whitehall since his request for British regiments was approved within days of arrival. In late December 1873 the first transports with British troops arrived off the coast, and in total more than 2,500 white soldiers were deployed against the Asante. From a military standpoint the campaign was a success, but from a medical point of view the outcome was more ambivalent. On the plus side the mortality rate was not excessive. Only 79 or 3 per cent of the white soldiers who arrived on the coast perished, with 17 of them being killed in action. The climate had not devastated the force, like many had feared, and this actually compared favourably with WIR soldiers who experienced a mortality rate of 3.7 per cent.[53] On the other hand, while Wolseley kept his promise of only retaining the white soldiers in the field for two months, 71 per cent of them fell sick during that period, leading him to conclude that a British empire in Africa 'does not come within the range of possible achievements'.[54] All the precautions he took to preserve the lives of white soldiers had worked, but he had not been able to prevent the climate nullifying his force fairly rapidly.

Anyone reading the published accounts of the Asante campaign, including Wolseley's own version published by his military secretary Henry Brackenbury, came away with two obvious conclusions. First, white soldiers could be used effectively for very short periods but were no long-term solution. And second, the WIRs were no better suited to African warfare. They succumbed to the same illness that prostrated the European soldier and were not as fit or robust as native levies. When Wolseley attempted to use WIR soldiers 'as carriers as a temporary measure', he found they 'were not so capable of doing work as the Fantis'.[55]

---

[52] Ibid., 303–4, 356. See also *The Star* (Guernsey), 23 August 1873.
[53] Ibid., 258–9.
[54] Brackenbury, *The Ashanti War*, II, 349–50.
[55] Ibid., II, 20, 23.

Despite his low opinion of the WIR soldiers as fighting men, Wolseley was not so foolish as to state that to the men themselves. On his departure from the Gold Coast in March 1874, he issued a general order expressing his appreciation of the 'soldier-like qualities' of the WIRs and acknowledging that they had 'undergone fatigue and exposure in a most creditable manner'.[56] The need to maintain morale among men who, after the European troops had departed, resumed their role as the sole British military force in the colony, was paramount. On their arrival back in Barbados, the 2WIR were feted with a grand public reception replete with speeches lauding the men's bravery.[57]

What had changed to make the WIR soldier so unsuited to African service? Surgeon Albert Gore, who had been stationed in West Africa during the 1860s and accompanied the Asante campaign in 1873–4, believed the reason to be the shifting nativity of WIR soldiers. Whereas formerly the men of the WIRs had been Africans, often recruited in Sierra Leone and shipped to the West Indies, by the 1860s the reverse was true. Most were now recruited locally in the West Indies and then rotated for a period of service in West Africa. Indeed, the change can readily be dated to the early 1850s since by 1853 Antiguans were complaining about the new practice of recruiting men for the 2WIR 'from the laborers of this island'.[58] Inevitably, Gore reported, since 'West Indian troops are alien to Africa; they consequently suffer more from climate than they would have done under the old system'.[59] From a medical standpoint Gore was right. Yellow fever was no longer endemic in the Caribbean by the second half of the nineteenth century, though it appeared periodically in epidemic form, and therefore WIR recruits would quite possibly not have been infected as children and so failed to gain the immunity their predecessors possessed. The defences those of West African origin possessed against malaria were genetic but did not protect against all the strains of the disease.[60]

Although Gore accepted Tulloch's argument that any transfer of soldiers from one climate to another, even if superficially similar, brought an increased risk of illness, he retained a belief that at least some sort

[56] A. B. Ellis, *The History of the First West India Regiment* (London: Chapman and Hall, 1885), 330.

[57] *Barbados Globe,* 11 May 1874.

[58] *Antigua Weekly Times,* 24 June 1853.

[59] Gore, *A Contribution to the Medical History,* 2.

[60] About 90 per cent of West Africans lack the Duffy antigen and are thus resistant to the vivax strain. Others had a degree of resistance to falciparum malaria via the 'sickle cell trait'. See Todd L. Savitt, *Medicine and Slavery: the Diseases and Healthcare of Blacks in Antebellum Virginia* (Urbana and Chicago: University of Illinois Press, 1981), 26–7.

of seasoning was possible. He recommended that a period of acclimation was required before a West Indian corps would be fully ready for service in West Africa, and he was not surprised when 'the left wing of the 4th, composed of a number of young men recently enlisted in the West Indies, suffered much on arrival from fever, owing to that want of habitual residence which appeared necessary to acclimatize the newly-arrived negro'.[61] Whether WIR soldiers would ever become as acclimated as native inhabitants was more open to doubt. Fellow surgeon Marcus Allen observed that West Africa was 'not inimical to the white man alone, but is also unsuited for any other than its own native inhabitants. This was remarkably exemplified during the late disturbance, in which the West India Regiments proved equally obnoxious to climatic influences with the European troops; so designedly does the land appear to have been made for the people, and the people for the land'.[62] Gore agreed that 'the West Indian soldiers became much more sickly on being transferred to the Coast of Africa, ... [and] the prevalence of constitutional affections in the Negro is strikingly shown, as well as the increase in febrile diseases and diseases of the digestive system on the change of station in the Negro'.[63] However, once the WIR soldiers had been in Africa for a while and survived 'the ordinary seasoning fever', they became, in Gore's view, 'much hardier and more capable of withstanding the effects of climate'.[64] The difference was one of degree. WIR soldiers were healthier than they had been on first arrival even if they could never match the health of local inhabitants.

James Africanus Horton, one of two African army surgeons serving in West Africa, thought the work of some of his eminent predecessors who had written on race and disease was deeply flawed. He was highly critical of those such as William Fergusson and Robert Jackson who had claimed that Africans were 'fever-proof', claims that were repeated and reprinted in the early nineteenth century until they became virtually unquestioned.[65] In his experience 'the African, especially the West Indian black of the present age, when exposed to the influence of malaria, suffers dreadfully from it, especially when brought in contact with it in a strange country'. During the Asante campaign nearly half the WIR troops stationed on the frontier reported sick with fever.

[61] Gore, *A Contribution to the Medical History*, 11.
[62] Marcus Allen, *The Gold Coast; or, a Cruise in West African Waters* (London: Hodder and Stoughton, 1874), 147.
[63] Ibid., 65.
[64] Ibid., 148.
[65] William Fergusson, 'On malaria and yellow fever in the West Indies', *United Service Journal* (1837), pt 3, 382.

While Horton, along with most others, accepted that WIR soldiers 'are not so susceptible as Europeans', something that justified their continued postings to Africa, the fact remained that 'their constitutions are by no means proof against its ravaging effects'.[66]

Reflecting in 1888's 'The negro as a soldier', Wolseley joined with Clarke and Gore in arguing that the fundamental shift in the ethnic origin of the WIRs during the nineteenth century had not been a positive development. Those purchased directly from slave ships, or recruited from intercepted slave ships after 1807, were 'fairly good fighting material.... They had a good physique,... could bear fatigue,... [were] brave, absolutely obedient... [and] possessed the best qualities which go to make up a really good soldier'. Since Wolseley never served in the Caribbean and did not commence his army career until the 1850s, he most likely gained this impression from reading published accounts, many of which were authored by surgeons such as William Fergusson and Robert Jackson, discussed in Chapter 2. The gradual suppression of the slave trade during the first half of the nineteenth century had meant that by 1860 'we can no longer obtain the wild negro from the interior of Africa', and as a result recruits were largely drawn from the West Indian islands, men whose immediate forebears had been enslaved. Previously 'each man could tell you the tribe on the West Coast to which he belonged.... Now the West Indian soldier will tell you he is a Barbadian, an Antiguan, a Jamaican, and so on'. Wolseley did not think this was a positive development since 'a large proportion of them have an infusion of white blood, which, strange to say, does not improve them physically'. Instead of their former robustness, Wolseley believed that white blood made these men vulnerable to the same diseases that affected whites and in West Africa this was a recipe for disaster.[67]

Wolseley rightly recalled that the entire justification for using the WIRs in Africa was their heightened ability to resist tropical diseases, and 'when these regiments were chiefly composed of Africans we had no trouble with them on the score of health, but now that they are raised from a class of negroes with a considerable portion of English blood in their veins they stand the climate at Cape Coast Castle and in the neighbouring provinces little better than the white man'. Without true African blood, the black soldier had been deprived of 'his natural hardihood'.[68] The emphasis placed on blood is informative since

---

[66] Horton, *The Diseases of Tropical Climates and Their Treatment*, 22.
[67] Viscount Wolseley, 'The negro as a solider', *The Fortnightly Review* 50 (1888), 689–90.
[68] Ibid.

it reflected the shift in racial attitudes that had occurred since mid-century. Remember it was Nott who had asserted the primacy of blood, instead of skin, in providing protection from yellow fever. Faced with mixed-race populations in both the West Indies and the United States, those seeking to maintain white supremacy stressed the taint that even one drop of African blood could bring.[69] Physical appearance, and specifically skin colour, was no longer a reliable guide to racial origins. For Wolseley the situation was reversed. The pure-blood African had been useful to the army, the mixed-race West Indian was not since 'the infusion of white blood into the West Indian negro has certainly not improved his physical strength, whilst the education we have given him has certainly injured his fighting qualities'. Those, including Josiah Nott, who had railed against 'mulatto hybrids' as being physically weaker than either of their parent races, had clearly influenced Wolseley's opinion.

Some of the special medical qualities previously attributed to WIR soldiers were now transferred onto local Africans. Marcus Allen remarked that 'not only is the native constitution so robust in resisting the forces that ordinarily engender illness, but it is endowed with the most extraordinary recuperative powers, and this enables it to make a remarkably rapid convalescence from injury and disease'. This lauding of the 'extraordinary instances of physical superiority' is exactly what Benjamin Moseley had said about black soldiers nearly a century before.[70] Albert Gore readily accepted that locally recruited African soldiers 'will undoubtedly stand a malarial climate and a tropical sun better than white troops, as they are not subject to the more severe forms of malarial diseases or yellow fever', but set against that was his low opinion of the bravery and intelligence of Africans. The WIRs were viewed as little better. They might be considered 'steady in action', but they were 'constant grumblers, ... disliked African service and surroundings, and looked forward to a return to the West Indies'.[71] The publicity surrounding the medical vulnerability of the WIRs clearly influenced army physicians posted to West Africa in the later nineteenth century. The discharge rates for WIR soldiers classified as medically unfit rose consistently, and the proportion of new recruits that passed medical muster declined. Despite the obvious medical risks, Gore thought the best

[69] See, for example, Ariela J. Gross, 'Litigating whiteness: trials of racial determination in the nineteenth-century South', *The Yale Law Journal* 108 (1998), 109–88; Joel Williamson, *New People: Miscegenation and Mulattoes in the United States* (New York: Free Press, 1980).
[70] Allen, *Gold Coast*, 134–5.
[71] Gore, *A Contribution to the Medical History*, 66, 68–9.

option for British colonies in West Africa was a force of European troops backed by 'disciplined and irregular native auxiliaries'.[72] African-born James Horton agreed. Using native Africans as a local police force would be an improvement on 'the soldiers of the West Indian Regiments, who have no stamina for bush operations'.[73]

Authorities in London did not respond positively to these ideas, perhaps remembering the high costs paid by white regiments in the past. Indeed, while the concept of the superhuman black soldier had been thoroughly debunked by the 1860s, the idea that white soldiers were now somehow able to resist tropical diseases, and African ones in particular, had yet to be widely accepted despite Wolseley's best efforts to rehabilitate them. The *Broad Arrow* thought 'the statement that West Indian negroes are less suited by nature to combat with the climate of the West Coast than European troops is not to be heard with patience' and suspected, correctly, that few would be 'over-ready to assume the responsibility of acting practically upon what is as best put forth as a theory'.[74] When the 2WIR disembarked in Barbados in May 1874 after serving in Africa, the local papers noted ruefully that 11 of the 15 white officers who had set out with the regiment had not returned but had been 'invalided' from service.[75] The number of white troops stationed in West Africa before 1900 remained small, usually under a hundred men consisting mainly of the officers of the WIRs and companies of the Royal Artillery. The data sent back to London showed they continued to fall sick and die at twice the rate of black troops, so the caution of London authorities seemed to be justified.[76]

The negative reports of the performance of the WIRs in 1864 and again in 1873–4 undermined any lingering confidence in their military abilities. The reputation of the WIRs had been both forged and shattered by war. The war with France between 1795 and 1815 had created the idea of the superhuman black soldier. The war against the Asante thoroughly dismantled it. Although the WIRs remained the principal British military unit in the region for the rest of the nineteenth century, they would spend most of their time on garrison duty.[77]

---

[72] Ibid., 68–9; Curtin, 'African health at home and abroad', 377–8.

[73] J. A. B. Horton, *West African Countries and Peoples, British and Native* (London: John Churchill, 1868), 268.

[74] *Broad Arrow*, 3 January 1874, reprinted in *Barbados Globe,* 16 February 1874.

[75] *Barbados Times,* 9 May 1874.

[76] *Army Medical Department Report for the Year 1898* (London: HMSO, 1900), 122–3.

[77] On average about 500 WIR soldiers were stationed in West Africa in the 1880s, rising to nearly 1,000 in the 1890s.

The fact that the men of the WIRs proved more susceptible to tropical fevers than anyone had previously thought possible mattered little in the grand scheme of things. Nobody in London took much notice if the data showed sickness and mortality rates for the WIRs were higher than average. Their role was primarily to be a British military presence that would deter possible outside aggression. When active operations were needed, small numbers of white troops were dispatched to work in conjunction with native levies. The unique medical status afforded to the WIRs was clearly over.

Conclusion

By the start of the twentieth century, the medical rationale for having black soldiers as an integral part of the British army had entirely dissipated. In the 1790s the army had valued the WIRs most particularly for the men's resistance to tropical diseases that decimated white regiments. Without the yellow fever epidemic of 1793, there would quite possibly have never been a need for the WIRs. But as the WIRs transformed from being composed mainly of African-born men to Caribbean-born men, their immunological advantage had waned. By mid-century, just as polygenism reached its zenith, it was becoming increasingly apparent that WIR soldiers possessed little more resistance to tropical diseases in West Africa than white men. The most effective medical treatment for malaria, using quinine, was recommended for white troops in West Africa both as a treatment and as a prophylactic as early as 1848, though its systematic use was not apparent until the Asante campaign of 1873–4.[1] There is little evidence of quinine being administered to black troops before the end of the century. In 1881 'a large proportion of the West Indian N.C. officers and men were prostrated with fever' while stationed at Cape Coast Castle, and in 1891 more than half of hospital admissions among WIR troops serving in Africa were attributed to 'malarial fevers'.[2] By 1900 the Army Medical Department also knew that mosquitoes were the vector for tropical diseases, and they began to take preventative measures against the insect, including the elimination of standing or stagnant bodies of water used

[1] Philip D. Curtin, 'The end of the "white man's grave"? Nineteenth-century mortality in west Africa', *The Journal of Interdisciplinary History* 21 (1990), 74. Philip D. Curtin, *The Image of Africa: British Ideas and Action* (Madison: University of Wisconsin Press, 1964), 344–56.
[2] J. E. Caulfeild, *One Hundred Years' History of the 2nd Batt. West India Regiment* (London: Forster Groom, 1899), 184. *Army Medical Department Report for the Year 1891* (London: HMSO, 1893), 96. Philip D. Curtin, 'African health at home and abroad', *Social Science History* 10 (1986), 387.

for breeding and netting beds to prevent bites.[3] They also made a more concerted effort to improve freshwater supplies for the small numbers of white troops stationed in Africa, and they established efficient methods of repatriation for the sick. The result of all these measures was a rapid fall in white mortality even in West Africa.[4]

The WIRs persisted as regular units of the British army until 1927 because they remained useful as garrison troops in both the Caribbean and West Africa. Lieutenant General Sir Charles Pearson, who led the West India Command between 1885 and 1890, considered the WIRs under his command to be 'excellent colonial troops'. But despite affection for his 'big stout fellows', Pearson could not hide from the fact that 'they suffer more than the white man from pulmonary complaints'. Even yellow fever, never a real respecter of race, now 'attacked non-European, as well as European troops', and two WIR soldiers died of the disease in Jamaica in 1897.[5] But while yellow fever never entirely disappeared from the Caribbean, the outbreaks were now far more sporadic and usually localised. The medical crisis that had forced the army's hand in 1795, and sustained the need for black troops throughout much of the nineteenth century, was over. Indeed, such was the general improvement in military mortality by the end of the nineteenth century that Pearson believed 'many of these lovely islands have become health resorts'.[6] The comparative medical advantage previously enjoyed by black troops in the West Indies simply no longer held true.

In West Africa, despite the use of quinine and measures taken against mosquitoes, no one seriously contemplated a large permanent white force, and total reliance on local levies was out of the question. As one soldier witheringly put it, 'West African tribes are worse than useless as levies ... their natural cowardice will lead them, when the fight is going against them, to run away at the critical moment'.[7]

---

[3] Capt. F. Smith, 'The distribution of mosquito larvae on war department lands in Sierra Leone' *Army Medical Department Report for the Year 1900* (London: HMSO, 1902), 495–501; *Army Medical Department Report for the Year 1906* (London: HMSO, 1907), 117. The pioneering work linking malaria with mosquitoes was R. Ross, 'On some peculiar pigmented cells found in two mosquitoes fed on malarial blood', *British Medical Journal* 2 (1897), 1786–8.

[4] Curtin, 'The end of the "white man's grave"', 75–6.

[5] *Army Medical Department Report for the Year 1897* (London: HMSO, 1899), 106–7.

[6] Sir Charles Pearson. 'The West Indies and its command', *United Service Magazine* (1894), 150, 152, 157. See also Melissa Bennett, 'Picturing the West India regiments: race, empire, and photography c. 1850–1914', unpublished PhD dissertation, University of Warwick (2018), 257–61.

[7] *Journal of the Royal United Service Institute* (March 1896), cited in Robert Stephenson Smyth Baden-Powell, *The Downfall of Prempeh: a Diary of Life with the Native Levy in Ashanti, 1895–6* (London: Methuen and Co., 1898), 177.

Brigadier General James Willcocks, encountering the WIR for the first time near Lagos in 1898, considered them ideally suited to garrison duty, describing them as 'burly, well-built men, with plenty of physical strength and endurance'. It was vitally important, however, 'never to give the black man an idea that you seek his assistance against other white men', thus the only suitable military use for the black soldier, he counselled, was against other black soldiers.[8] During World War I the WIR proved its military worth once more, first in Cameroon, then in East Africa and finally in Palestine, winning battle honours for each campaign. Brigadier General Howard Gorges, leading the Cameroon campaign, was glad the army did not have to rely on native troops, believing 'the West Indian soldier was endowed with a higher intellect than the West African, and many of the men were well educated and intelligent, making first-class signallers and telephone operators. They were also well-disciplined, staunch troops and good shots'.[9] The fact that the men of the WIR spoke English and were accustomed to British military discipline bolstered confidence in their loyalty but, following Willcocks' advice, the WIR was never deployed against a white enemy.

The WIRs are clearly unusual. For more than forty years the majority view of these black soldiers was positive. Army commanders praised everything about them, from their legendary resistance to tropical illnesses to their impressive stamina and their bravery. Even when bumps in the road appeared, such as the mutiny in Dominica in 1802 that could easily have been used as an excuse to swiftly terminate the experiment with black soldiers, they were explained away: the men had been mistreated by their commanders, forced to do un-soldierly tasks and incorrectly paid. Nothing could be permitted to subvert the general opinion that in forming the WIRs the British army had taken a forward-thinking and sensible step. The positivity around the WIRs was not just about the black soldier, either individually or as a collective unit, it was also about blackness per se. Army surgeons told anyone who would listen that WIR soldiers owed their medical superiority over whites to their black skin, and they made little distinction between recruits born in the West Indies, North America, West Africa or East Africa. Quite simply, there are few comparable examples of black people in the nineteenth century being considered in such a positive light.

---

[8] James Willcocks, *From Kabul to Kumassi: Twenty-Four Years of Soldiering and Sport* (London: John Murray, 1904), 194–5.

[9] Howard Gorges, *The Great War in West Africa* (London: Naval and Military Press, 2004), 43.

In the early nineteenth century, slavery remained the paradigm by which most British people defined black people. The vast majority of published works in English between 1780 and 1865 that mentioned those of African descent concerned either the system of enslavement in the West Indies or the American South or the slave trade. Those campaigning to abolish first the transatlantic slave trade, and then slavery as a system, made their case largely on humanitarian and religious grounds, that owning other people was immoral and mistreating them was worse. Few made a case for a more positive view of the black body, one that might hold special qualities lacking in white people. In fact, the opposite was the case, with those defending slavery praising the ability of the enslaved to labour in tropical heat. When emancipation came there was little effort made to treat former slaves as the political or social equals of whites, and concerted efforts were made to sustain old racial hierarchies. Yet army surgeons and commanders did not permit the wider denigration of black people in the Caribbean to shape their own views. The WIRs, as far as they were concerned, were full of strong, capable men, especially suited, both medically and physically, to a military life. Their supposedly inferior intellectual capabilities were also viewed in a positive light since no commander wanted soldiers who thought for themselves. Instead obedience to orders and the ability to follow direction were prioritised.

Confidence in the special medical abilities of the WIR went largely unchallenged until Alexander Tulloch began to work with the statistics gathered by the Army Medical Board. Tulloch planted the seed of doubt about the superhuman nature of black skin. In fact, it was more than a seed of doubt, rather a forest of seedlings. In the 1850s polygenists like Josiah Nott took these seedlings of doubt, fed, watered and propagated them, so they became more than doubts and were now fully grown facts that not only undermined the special properties of black skin but also questioned the right of black people to even count as members of the human race. Polygenists took what previously had been seen as a positive, that black bodies were different from white bodies, and transformed it into something highly negative. Any permanent physical differences would have sufficed in their drive to deny the unity of the human species; the fact that Tulloch had helpfully stressed the vulnerability of the black body to certain diseases was an added bonus. Polygenism waxed and waned comparatively quickly but left behind a permanent intellectual legacy emphasising black medical inferiority. What finally killed off the idea of the medically superior black soldier was the Asante campaign of 1873–4, the most prominent and well-publicised British military effort in West Africa in the nineteenth century. No longer did those denigrating the black military body have to rely on dry statistics or ethnological theory – they had evidence from well-respected army commanders confirming that black soldiers were just as vulnerable to tropical illnesses as white soldiers, and they failed to match the latter's bravery, intelligence and military skill.

The generally negative image of the WIRs that emerged and persisted during the second half of the nineteenth century both reflected and reinforced contemporary notions about blackness. Slavery might have ended in the British Caribbean in 1838 and in the United States in 1865, but ideas about black inferiority were so entrenched that emancipation was never going to lead to true equality. Former slave owners maintained or re-established political control in the West Indies and the American South, and they invented new ways to marginalise and suppress the emancipated black population. In Britain, where the black population had always been comparatively tiny, ideas about blackness (or perhaps non-whiteness is a better way to look at it) were more likely to be influenced by imperialism. The second half of the nineteenth century saw Britain expand its empire in western, southern and eventually eastern Africa, as well as south Asia. Accounts of military success against far less technologically advanced non-white peoples appeared in the press, helping to confirm the superiority of British (i.e. white) civilisation in the popular imagination. Most of the time imperial expansion was achieved by white troops, or native troops under white officers.[10]

The history of the WIRs is therefore a mirror of how black people more generally were treated in the nineteenth century. But racist denigration was far more than something simply done to, or experienced by, the WIRs. The men themselves provided the empirical and statistical evidence that shaped racial thought. Without the WIRs Tulloch would not have been able to make his sweeping claims about black bodies, and those claims would not have been picked up and subsequently magnified by the polygenists. Without surgeons treating and studying the men of the WIRs, the knowledge of the black male body would have remained fragmented and largely shaped by slavery. The medical data suggest that the vulnerability of black soldiers to disease did not actually change that radically during the nineteenth century. Sickness rates were perhaps a little higher overall in the second half of the nineteenth century, but mortality rates remained fairly stable and even fell slightly. The significant improvement came in white sickness and mortality, brought

[10] See, for example, Brian Bond, *Victorian Military Campaigns* (London: Hutchinson, 1967); Bruce Vandervort, *Wars of Imperial Conquest in Africa, 1830–1914* (Bloomington: Indiana University Press, 1998), 113–84.

about by a combination of reforms to accommodation, diet, rotation schedules and medical care.[11] The inability of the black soldier to match the improvements for his white counterpart was most often blamed on inherent weaknesses of black male bodies, rather than on external factors that were entirely under the army's control.

The achievements of the WIRs were considerable. In purely military terms it is quite likely that the history of the West Indies and West Africa would have been very different without them. Revolutionary sentiments emerging from French Caribbean islands in the 1790s could easily have spread to British islands, leading to either more independent black republics, along the lines of Haiti, or loose French oversight. In West Africa the absence of a permanent garrison of British troops would almost certainly have emboldened African kingdoms to continuously test British resolve. The British Empire would have been smaller and weaker without the WIRs. The same is true of medical literature about tropical diseases and about blackness. Without the WIRs most writers would have had little to work with, and certainly nothing like the detailed records that were generated by the WIRs. In both military and medical terms, the men of the WIRs proved to be some of the most important men of African descent in the Atlantic World.

---

[11] Curtin, *Image of Africa*, 344–56; John Rankin, *Healing the African Body: British Medicine in West Africa, 1800–1860* (Columbia: University of Missouri Press, 2015), 131.

Bibliography

MSS Sources

British Library, London

Correspondence of the 5th Duke of Leeds v.3, 1787 Add MS 28062 (f.378)
Abstract of British West Indian Trade and Navigation from 1773 to 1805 Stowe 921
Lady Nugent's Journal – Jamaica one hundred and thirty-eight years ago W6/9664
Sir John Moore Papers 17 November 1796 – 24 October 1797 Add MS 57327

University College, London

West India Committee Archives (microfilm)

Wellcome Library, London

Observations and remarks on the quarterly returns of sick of the troops serving on the Island of St Vincent RAMC 397/B/RR/1
Correspondence on the Regalia RAMC 212/36

Library of Congress

E. G. Squier Papers

The National Archives, Kew, London

Colonial Office
CO28/85–97 Barbados
CO71/29–34 Dominica
CO91/44 and 58 Gibraltar
CO92/4 Gibraltar

CO101/31–34 Grenada
CO137/88–145 Jamaica
CO267/49–50 and 91 Sierra Leone
CO295/114–5 Trinidad
CO318/19–54 Dispatches
CO318/128 Letters
CO320/3 Report on black troops, 1836

War Office

WO1/31–2 Martinique
WO1/59–69 St Domingue
WO1/83–90 Windward Islands
WO1/92 Letters
WO1/93 Trinidad
WO1/95–6 Dispatches
WO1/141 New Orleans
WO1/351 Africa
WO1/647 Correspondence 1811
WO4/158 Correspondence 1795
WO4/729 Correspondence 1836
WO17/1988–90 Jamaica returns
WO17/2486–94 Windward Islands returns
WO25/644–62 Succession books
WO25/2740 4WIR returns
WO27/90–147 Inspection reports
WO33/13 Memorandum on British possessions in West Africa
WO43/149 Royal African Corps
WO71/109 and 193 Courts martial
WO90/1 Courts martial register
WO96/94 Sierra Leone
WO284/20–1 Gibraltar garrison orders
WO334/2–174 Medical reports

Medical Journals

British Annals of Medicine
British and Foreign Medical Review
Charleston Medical Journal
Edinburgh Medical and Surgical Journal
Jamaica Physical Journal
London Medical Physical Journal
London Medical Journal
Medico Chirurgical Review
New Orleans Medical and Surgical Journal
Southern Journal of Medical and Physical Sciences
Southern Medical and Surgical Journal
Southern Medical Reports

Printed Primary Sources

'A further account of the mutiny of the 8th West India Regiment', *United Service Magazine* (1851), pt 3, 399–401.

Allen, Marcus, *The Gold Coast; Or, a Cruise in West African Waters* (London: Hodder and Stoughton, 1874).

Amringe, William Frederick Van, *An Investigation of the Theories of the Natural History of Man* (New York: Baker and Scribner, 1848).

Army Medical Department Reports 1859–1900 (London: HMSO, various dates).

Armstrong, Robert, *The Influence of Climate and Other Agents on the Human Constitution* (London: Longman, 1843).

Astley, Philip, *Remarks on the Profession and Duty of a Soldier* (London: for the author, 1794).

Atkins, John, *A Voyage to Guinea, Brasil, and the West-Indies; In His Majesty's Ships, the Swallow and Weymouth* (London: Caesar Ward and Richard Chandler, 1735).

Bachman, John, *A Notice of the 'Types of Mankind'* (Charleston: James, Williams and Gitsinger, 1854).

Bachman, John, 'An examination of the characteristics of genera', *Charleston Medical Journal* 10 (1855), 201–22.

Baden-Powell, Robert Stephenson Smyth, *The Downfall of Prempeh: a Diary of Life with the Native Levy in Ashanti, 1895–6* (London: Methuen and Co., 1898).

Bancroft, Edward, *A Sequel to an Essay on the Yellow Fever* (London: J. Callow, 1817).

Bayley, Frederick William Naylor, *Four Years' Residence in the West Indies during the Years 1826, 7, 8 and 9 by the Son of a Military Officer* (London: William Kidd, 1833).

Beaver, Philip, *African Memoranda Relative to an Attempt to Establish a British Settlement on the Island of Bulama* (London: C. and R. Baldwin, 1805).

Bell, Andrew, *The Madras School* (London: T. Ensley, 1808).

Bell, John, *An Inquiry into the Causes Which Produce and the Means of Preventing Diseases among British Officers, Soldiers and Others in the West Indies* (London: J. Murray, 1791).

Benezet, Anthony, *Observations on the Inslaving, Importing and Purchasing of Negroes* (Germantown: Christopher Sower, 1759).

Benezet, Anthony, *Some Historical Account of Guinea* (Philadelphia: Joseph Crukshank, 1771).

Benezet, Anthony, *The Case of Our Fellow Creatures, the Oppressed Africans* (London: James Phillips, 1784).

Bigland, John, *Historical Display of the Effects of Physical and Moral Causes on the Character and Circumstances of Nations* (London: Longman, 1816).

Blair, Daniel, *Report on the First Eighteen Months of the Fourth Yellow Fever Epidemic of British Guiana* (London: Savill and Edwards, Printers, 1856).

Blair, Daniel, *Some Account of the Last Yellow Fever Epidemic of British Guiana* (London: Longman, Brown, Green and Longmans, 1850).

Brackenbury, Henry, *The Ashanti War: a Narration Prepared from the Official Documents* (Edinburgh: William Blackwood, 1874).

Buisseret, David, *Jamaica in 1687: the Taylor Manuscript at the National Library Jamaica* (Kingston, Jamaica: University of the West Indies Press, 2000).

Burke, Edmund, *An Account of the European Settlements in America* (London: R. J. Dodsley, 1760).

Burton, E. J., 'Observations on the climate, topography, and diseases of the British colonies in western Africa', *Provincial Medical and Surgical Journal* 3 (1842), 249–51; 265–6; 287–90; 306–9; 323–6; 346–9; 365–8; 392–5.

Caldwell, Charles, *Thoughts on the Original Unity of the Human Race* (New York: E. Bliss, 1830).

Campbell, John, *Negro-mania: Being an Examination of the Falsely Assumed Equality of the Various Races of Men* (Philadelphia: Campbell and Power, 1851).

Cartwright, Samuel, 'Diseases and peculiarities of the negro race', *De Bow's Review* 9 (1851), 64–9.

Cartwright, Samuel, 'Report on the diseases and physical peculiarities of the negro race', *Southern Medical Reports* 2 (1850), 421–9.

Cartwright, Samuel, 'Statistical medicine or numerical analysis applied to the investigation of morbid actions', *Western Journal of Medicine and Surgery* 1 (1848), 185–206.

Caulfeild, James E., *One Hundred Years' History of the 2nd Batt. West India Regiment* (London: Forster Groom, 1899).

Chisholm, Colin, *An Essay on the Malignant Pestilential Fever Introduced into the West Indian Islands from Boullam, on the Coast of Guinea, as It Appeared in 1793 and 1794* (London: C. Dilly, 1795 and Philadelphia: Thomas Dobson, 1799).

Clark, James, *A Treatise on the Yellow Fever as It Appeared in the Island of Dominica in the Years 1793–4–5–6* (London: J. Murray, 1797).

Clark, James, *A Treatise on Tubercular Phthisis* (London: Marchant, 1834).

Coles, Abraham, *A Critique on Nott and Gliddon's Ethnological Works* (Burlington: Medical and Surgical Reporter, 1857).

Combe, George, *The Constitution of Man* (Edinburgh: John Anderson, 1828, reprinted Cambridge University Press, 2009).

Dancer, Thomas, *A Brief History of the Late Expedition against Fort San Juan, So Far as It Relates to the Diseases of the Troops* (Kingston, Jamaica: D. Douglass and W. Aikman, 1781).

Darwin, Charles, *On the Origin of Species by Means of Natural Selection* (London: John Murray, 1859).

Darwin, Charles, *The Descent of Man and Selection in Relation to Sex* (London: John Murray, 1871).

Dickinson, Nodes, *Observations on the Inflammatory Endemic Incidental to Strangers in the West Indies from Temperate Climates Commonly Called the Yellow Fever* (London: E. Hewlett, 1819).

Dirom, Alex, *Thoughts on the State of the Militia of Jamaica Nov 1783* (Kingston, Jamaica: D. Douglass and W. Aikman, 1783).

Dodd, Charles R., *The Annual Biography* (London: Chapman and Hall, 1843).

Dundas, Henry, *Facts Relative to the Conduct of the War in the West Indies* (London: J. Owen, 1796).

Edwards, Bryan, *An Historical Survey of the French Colony in the Island of St Domingo* (London: John Stockdale, 1797).

Edwards, Bryan, *The History, Civil and Commercial of the British Colonies in the West Indies* (London: John Stockdale, 1801).

Ellis, Alfred Burdon, *The History of the First West India Regiment* (London: Chapman and Hall Ltd, 1885).

Equiano, Olaudah, *The Interesting Life of Olaudah Equiano or Gustavus Vassa, the African* (London: for the author, 1789).

Fellowes, Sir James, *Reports of the Pestilential Disorder of Andalusia* (London: Longman, 1815).

Fenner, E. D., 'Acclimation; and the liability of negroes to the endemic fevers of the south', *Southern Medical and Surgical Journal* 14 (1858), 452–60.

Fergusson, William, 'An inquiry into the origin and nature of the yellow fever', *Medico Chirurgical Transactions* 8 (1817), 108–72.

Fergusson, William, 'Dr Fergusson on Yellow Fever', *Medico Chirurgical Review* 32 (1840), 297–307.

Fergusson, William, 'Dr Fergusson's remarks on the statistical report on the sickness &c among the troops in the West Indies', *United Service Journal* (1838), pt 3, 235–40.

Fergusson, William, *Notes and Recollections of a Professional Life* (London: Longman, 1846).

Fergusson, William, 'On barrack accommodation in the West Indies', *United Service Journal* (1838), pt 1, 89–96.

Fergusson, William, 'On malaria and yellow fever in the West Indies', *United Service Journal* (1837), pt 3, 377–82.

Fergusson, William, 'On the qualities and employment of black troops in the West Indies', *United Service Journal* (1835), pt 1, 523–8.

Fergusson, William, 'On the supposed contagious property of yellow fever', *United Service Journal* (1838), pt 2, 380–5.

Forbes, John, Alexander Tweedie and John Conolly (eds.), *The Cyclopaedia of Practical Medicine* (London: Sherwood, Gilbert and Piper, 1835).

Forwood, W. S., 'The negro – a distinct species', *Medical and Surgical Reporter* 10 (1857), 225–35.

Fourth Report of the Directors of the African Institution (London: J. Hatchard, 1810).

Fowle, William, *A Practical Treatise on the Different Fevers of the West Indies* (London: H. D. Symonds, 1800).

Gillespie, Leonard, *Observations on the Diseases Which Prevailed on Board a Part of His Majesty's Squadron on the Leeward Island Station between Nov. 1794 and April 1796* (London: G. Auld, 1800).

Gilpin, Joseph, 'Remarks on the fever which occurred at Gibraltar in 1813', *Edinburgh Medical and Surgical Journal* 10 (1814), 311–17.

Gobineau, Joseph A. (Josiah Nott, trans.), *The Moral and Intellectual Diversity of Races* (Philadelphia: J. Lippincott, 1856).

Gordon, John, *Proceedings of the General Court Martial in the Trial of Major J. Gordon, of the late 8th West India Regiment* (London: E. Lloyd, 1804).

Gore, Albert A., *A Contribution to the Medical History of Our West African Campaign* (London: Bailliere, Tindall and Cox, 1876).

Goupil, J. M. A. (J. Nott, trans.), *An Exposition on the Principles of the New Medical Doctrine* (Columbia, SC: Times and Gazette Office, 1831).

Halliday, Sir Andrew, *A Letter to the Right Honourable, the Secretary at War, on Sickness and Mortality in the West Indies: Being a Review of Captain Tulloch's Statistical Report* (London: John Parker, 1839).

Halliday, Sir Andrew, *The West Indies: the Natural and Physical History of the Windward and Leeward Colonies* (London: John William Parker, 1837).

Hamilton, Ronald, *Sketch of the Present State of the Army* (London: J. Owen, 1796).

Hamilton, Robert, *The Duties of a Regimental Surgeon Considered* (London: J. Johnson, 1787).

Harvey, W. M. and John Lindesay, 'Account of the cachexia Africana: a disease incidental to negro slaves lately imported into the West Indies', *The Medical Repository of Original Essays and Intelligence* 2 (1799), 281–4.

Hennen, John, *Sketches of the Medical Topography of the Mediterranean* (London: Thomas and George Underwood, 1830).

Hillary, William, *Observations on the Changing Nature of the Air and the Concomitant Epidemical Diseases in the Island of Barbadoes*, 2nd ed. (London: L. Hawes, 1766).

Horton, James Africanus B., *The Diseases of Tropical Climates and Their Treatment* (London: J. and A. Churchill, 1874).

Horton, James Africanus B., *West African Countries and Peoples, British and Native* (London: John Churchill, 1868).

Hughes, Griffith, *Natural History of Barbados* (London: Author, 1750).

Hunt, James, 'On ethno-climatology; Or the acclimatization of man', *Transactions of the Ethnological Society of London* 2 (1863), 50–83.

Hunt, Sanford B., 'The negro as a soldier', *Quarterly Journal of Psychological Medicine* 1 (1867), 1661–86.

Hunter, John, *Observations on the Diseases of the Army in Jamaica* (London: G. Nicol, 1788).

Jackson, Robert, *A Sketch of the History and Cure of Febrile Diseases; More Particularly as They Appear in the West Indies among Soldiers of the British Army* (Stockton: T. and H. Eeles, 1817).

Jackson, Robert, *A Treatise on the Fevers of Jamaica, with Some Observations on the Intermitting Fever of America* (London: J. Murray, 1791).

Jackson, Robert, *An Outline of the History and Cure of Fever, Endemic and Contagious* (Edinburgh: Mundell and Son, 1798).

James, Charles, *The Regimental Companion* (London: T. Egerton, 1800).

Johnstone, Andrew, *Defence of the Honourable Andrew Cochrane Johnstone* (Edinburgh: Manners and Miller, 1806).

Kames, Henry, *Sketches of the History of Man in Two Volumes* (Edinburgh: W. Creech, 1774).

Knox, Robert, *Races of Men: a Fragment* (Philadelphia: Lea and Blanchard, 1850).

Lawrence, William, *Lectures on Physiology, Zoology, and the Natural History of Man* (London: J. Callow, 1819).

Lawson, Robert, 'Observations on the outbreak of yellow fever among the troops at Newcastle, Jamaica, in the latter part of 1856', *British Foreign Medical Review* 24 (1859), 324–49.

Lawson, Thomas, *Statistical Report on the Sickness and Mortality in the Army of the United States* (Washington, DC: Jacob Gideon, 1840).

Lempriere, William, *Practical Observations on the Diseases of the Army in Jamaica as they Occurred between the Years 1792 and 1797* (London: T. N. Longman, 1799).

Letter of an Old Field Officer on Military Punishments (London: for the author, 1837).

Ligon, Richard, *A True and Exact History of the Island of Barbadoes* (London: Humphrey Moseley, 1657).

Lind, James, *An Essay on Diseases Incidental to Europeans in Hot Climates* (London: T. Beckett, 1768).

Long, Edward, *The History of Jamaica* (London: T. Lowndes, 1774).

Mackellar, Patrick, *A Correct Journal of the Landing His Majesty's Forces on the Island of Cuba; And of the Siege and Surrender of the Havannah, August 13, 1762* (London, Green and Russell, 1762).

M'Cabe, James, *Military Medical Reports: Containing Pathological and Practical Observations Illustrating the Diseases of Warm Climates* (Cheltenham: G. A. Williams, 1825).

M'Lean, Hector, *An Enquiry into the Nature, and Causes of the Great Mortality among the Troops at St Domingo: with Practical Remarks on the Fever of That Island; And Directions, for the Conduct of Europeans on Their First Arrival in Warm Climates* (London: T. Cadell, 1797).

M'Lean, Hector, 'Man's power of adaptation to different climates', *Pennsylvania Journal of Prison Discipline and Philanthropy* 5 (1850), 5–15.

Marshall, Henry, 'A historical sketch of military punishments, in as far as regards non-commissioned officers and private soldiers', *United Service Journal* (1843), pt 2, 63–70; 234–40; 384–95; 520–30; (1843), pt 3, 104–14; 385–99; 558–68; (1844), pt 1, 70–76; 242–56; 410–16; (1844), pt 2, 82–88; 251–8.

Marshall, Henry, 'Contribution to statistics of the army with some observations on military medical returns', *The Edinburgh Medical and Surgical Journal* 40 (1833), 36–44; 307–21.

Marshall, Henry, *Military Miscellany* (London: John Murray, 1846).

Marshall, Henry, *Notes on the Medical Topography of the Interior of Ceylon* (London: Burgess and Hill, 1821).

Martin, W. C. Linnaeus, *A General Introduction to the Natural History of Mammiferous Animals* (London: Wright and Co., 1841).

Mathew, Captain, 'Four years on the Gold Coast', *United Service Magazine* (1864), pt 2, 272–6; 371–83; 541–53; pt 3, 47–59.

Maurice, J. F., *The Diary of Sir John Moore* (London: Edward Arnold, 1904).

Moore, Francis, *Travels into the Inland Parts of Africa* (London: Edward Cave, 1738).

Morton, Samuel, *Brief Remarks on the Diversities of the Human Species* (Philadelphia: Merrihew and Thompson, 1842).

Morton, Samuel, *Illustrations of Pulmonary Consumption* (Philadelphia: Key and Biddle, 1834).

Moseley, Benjamin, *A Treatise on Tropical Diseases on Military Operations*, 2nd ed. (London: T. Cadell, 1789).

Nott, Josiah C., *An Essay on the Natural History of Mankind Viewed in Connection with Negro Slavery* (Mobile: Dade, Thompson and Co., 1851).

Nott, Josiah C., 'Geographical distribution of animals and the races of men', *New Orleans Medical and Surgical Journal* 9 (1853), 727–46.

Nott, Josiah C., *Instincts of Races* (New Orleans: L. Graham, 1866).

Nott, Josiah C., 'Statistics of southern slave populations', *De Bow's Commercial Review of the South and West* 2 (1847), 275–89.

Nott, Josiah C., 'The mulatto a hybrid', *Boston Medical and Surgical Journal* 29 (1843), 29–32.

Nott, Josiah C., 'The negro race', *Popular Magazine of Anthropology* 1 (1866), 102–18.

Nott, Josiah C., *Two Lectures on the Natural History of the Caucasian and Negro Races* (Mobile: Dade and Thompson, 1844).

Nott, Josiah C., 'Unity of the human race', *Southern Quarterly Review* 9 (1846), 1–57.

Nott, Josiah C., 'Yellow fever contrasted with bilious fever', *New Orleans Medical and Surgical Journal* 4 (1848), 563–601.

Nott, Josiah C. and George R. Gliddon, *Indigenous Races of the Earth* (Philadelphia: Lippincott and Co., 1857).

Nott, Josiah C. and George R. Gliddon, *Types of Mankind* (Philadelphia: Lippincott, Grambo and Co., 1854).

O'Connor, Luke Smyth, 'Leaves from the tropics', *United Service Journal* (1848), pt 1, 329–40; pt 2, 347–57; pt 3, 55–69; 209–17; (1849), pt 1, 110–21; pt 2, 520–35; pt 3, 56–77; 223–30.

O'Connor, Luke Smyth, 'On the military defences and "expenditure" of the West Indies', *United Service Journal* (1851), pt 3, 161–71.

O'Connor, Luke Smyth, 'Suggestions for the discipline, uniform, messing and recruiting of the West India Regiments', *United Service Journal* (1837), pt 1, 361–6.

O'Connor, Luke Smyth, 'The command in the Windward and Leeward islands', *United Service Journal* (1843), pt 2, 89–102.

O'Connor, Luke Smyth, 'Twelve months service in Western Africa' (1845), pt 2, 57–70; 235–44; 424–32; 587–95; pt 3, 196–210; 505–13; (1846), pt 1, 217–27.

Ogilby, John, *Africa, Being an Accurate Description of the Regions* (London: Tho. Johnson, 1670).

Ogilby, John, 'On the utility and economy of the West India Regiments', *United Service Journal* (1833), pt 2, 492–6.

Ogilby, John, 'Our military establishments in the West Indies', *United Service Journal* (1866), pt 1, 244–7.

Pearson, Charles, 'The West Indies and its command', *United Service Magazine* (1894), 150–7.

Pinckard, George, *Notes on the West Indies* (London: Baldwin, Cradock and Joy, 1816).

Poyer, John, *The History of Barbados from the First Discovery of the Island* (London: J. Mawman, 1808).

Prichard, James Cowles, *Researches into the Physical History of Man* (London: John and Arthur Arch, 1813).

Priest, Josiah, *Slavery, as It Relates to the Negro, or African Race* (Louisville: W. S. Brown, 1849).

Pym, William, *Observations on Bulam Fever Which Has of Late Years Prevailed in the West Indies, on the Coast of America, at Gibraltar, Cadiz and Other Parts of Spain* (London: J. Callow, 1815).

Pym, William, *Observations on Bulam, Vomito-negro or Yellow Fever* (London: John Churchill, 1848).

Ramsay, H. A., *The Necrological Appearances of Southern Typhoid Fever in the Negro* (Columbia Co. GA: Constitutionalist Office, 1852).

Ramsay, W. G., 'The physiological differences between the European (or white man) and the negro', *Southern Agriculturalist* 12 (1839), 412–18.

Rankin, F. Harrison, *The White Man's Grave: a Visit to Sierra Leone in 1834* (London: Richard Bentley, 1836).

'Reflections on recent events in Jamaica', *United Service Magazine* (1866), pt 2, 100–13; 196–209.

Reece, Richard, *The Medical Guide for Tropical Climates* (London: Longman, Hurst, Reese, Orme and Brown, 1814).

Reide, Thomas Dickson, *A View of the Diseases of the Army in Great Britain, America, the West-Indies and On Board of King's Ships and Transports* (London: J. Johnson, 1793).

Roche, R. La, 'Remarks on the connection, pathological and etiological, supposed to exist between pneumonia and periodic fever', *Charleston Medical Journal*, 8 (1853), 577–82.

Smith, Charles Hamilton, *Costumes of the Army of the British Empire* (London: Colnaghi and Co., 1812).

Smith, Charles Hamilton, *The Natural History of the Human Species* (Boston: Gould and Lincoln, 1851).

Smith, Samuel Stanhope, *Essay on the Causes of the Variety of Complexion and Figure in the Human Species* (Philadelphia: Robert Aitken, 1787).

Smythson, Hugh, *The Compleat Family Physician or, Universal Medical Repository* (London: Harrison and Co., 1785).

Southey, Thomas, *Chronological History of the West Indies* (London: Longman, 1827).

Stephen, James, *Slavery in the British West India Colonies Delineated* (London: Joseph Butterworth, 1824).

Stewart, J., *A View of the Past and Present State of the Island of Jamaica: with Remarks on the Moral and Physical Condition of the Slaves and the Abolition of Slavery in the Colonies* (Edinburgh: Oliver and Boyd, 1823).

'The mutiny of the 8th West India Regiment from the papers of a veteran officer', *United Service Magazine* (1851), pt 3, 207–10.

'The West India Regiments and the defence of the colonies', *United Service Magazine* (1865), pt 1, 211–17.

Thomson, James, *A Treatise on the Diseases of Negroes as They Occur in the Island of Jamaica* (Jamaica: Alex Aikman, 1820).

Thomson, Arthur S., 'Could the natives of a temperate climate colonize and increase in a tropical country and vice versa?' *Transactions of the Medical and Physical Society of Bombay* 6 (1843), 112–38.

Thomson, Arthur S., 'On the doctrine of acclimatization', *Madras Quarterly Medical Journal* 2 (1840), 69–76.

Thomson, Arthur S., *On the Influence of Climate on the Health and Mortality of the Inhabitants of the Different Regions of the Globe* (Edinburgh: John Carfrae and Sons, 1837).

Towne, Richard, *A Treatise of the Diseases Most Frequent in the West Indies* (London: John Clarke, 1726).

Tuckey, James Hingston, *Narrative of an Expedition to Explore the River Zaire, Usually Called the Congo, in South Africa, in 1816* (London: J. Murray, 1818).

Tulloch, Alexander M., 'Observations on military pensions, and calculations of their value', *United Service Journal* (1835), pt 1, 145–79.

Tulloch, Alexander M., 'On the mortality among Her Majesty's troops serving in the colonies during the years 1844 and 1845', *Journal of the Statistical Society* 10 (1847), 252–9.

Tulloch, Alexander M., 'On the mortality among officers of the British army', *United Service Journal* (1835), pt 2, 145–72.

Tulloch, Alexander M., 'On the relief of corps on foreign service', *United Service Journal* (1836), pt 3, 289–305.

Tulloch, Alexander M., 'On the statistics of the negro slave population in the West Indies', *British Annals of Medicine* 13 and 15 (1837), 392–6; 449–54.

Tulloch, Alexander M., *Statistical Report on the Sickness, Mortality and Invaliding among the Troops in the West Indies; Prepared from the Records of the Army Medical Department and War-Office Returns* (London: W. Clowes and Sons, 1838).

Tulloch, Alexander M., *Statistical Reports on the Sickness, Mortality and Invaliding among the Troops in the United Kingdom, the Mediterranean and British America* (London: HM Stationery Office, 1839).

Tulloch, Alexander M., *Statistical Report on the Sickness, Mortality and Invaliding among the Troops in Western Africa, St Helena, the Cape of Good Hope and the Mauritius; Prepared from the Records of the Army Medical Department and War-Office Returns* (London: W. Clowes and Sons, 1840).

Tulloch, Alexander M., *Statistical Report on the Sickness, Mortality and Invaliding among Her Majesty's Troops Serving in Ceylon, the Tenasserim Provinces and the Burmese Empire; Prepared from the Records of the Army Medical Department and War-Office Returns* (London: W. Clowes and Sons, 1841).

Vandell, Lunsford P., 'Remarks on struma Africana, or the disease usually called negro poison or negro consumption', *Transylvania Journal of Medicine and Associate Sciences* 4 (1831), 83–103.

Virey, J-J. (J. H. Guenebault, trans.), *Natural History of the Negro Race* (Charleston: D. J. Dowling, 1837).

Warren, Henry, *A Treatise Concerning the Malignant Fever in Barbados* (London: Fletcher Gyles, 1740).

Wesley, John, *Thoughts upon Slavery* (London: R. Haws, 1774).

White, Charles, *An Account of the Regular Gradation in Man* (London: C. Dilly, 1799).

Willcocks, James, *From Kabul to Kumassi: Twenty-four Years of Soldiering and Sport* (London: John Murray, 1904).

Williams, Philip C., 'On acclimation', *The Medical Examiner and Record of Medical Science* 68 (1850), 447.

Williamson, John, *Medical and Miscellaneous Observations Relative to the West India Islands* (Edinburgh: Alex Smellie, 1817).

Wilson, Alexander, *Some Observations Relative to the Influence of Climate on Vegetables and Animal Bodies* (London: T. Cadell, 1780).

Wolseley, Viscount, 'The negro as a solider', *The Fortnightly Review* 50 (1888), 689–90.

Wright, William, *Memoir of the Late William Wright* (Edinburgh: William Blackwood, 1828).

Wright, William, 'Practical observations on the treatment of acute diseases, particularly those of the West Indies', *Medical Facts and Observations* 7 (1797), 8–9.

Woods, Joseph, *Thoughts on the Slavery of the Negroes* (London: for the author, 1788).

Young, Sir William, *The West-India Common-Place Book* (London: Richard Phillips, 1807).

Secondary Sources

Ackroyd, Marcus, Laurence Brockliss, Michael Moss, Kate Retford, and John Stevenson, *Advancing with the Army: Medicine, the Professions, and Social Mobility in the British Isles, 1790–1850* (Oxford: Oxford University Press, 2006).

Alsop, J. D., 'Warfare and the creation of British imperial medicine, 1600–1800', in G. Hudson (ed.), *British Military and Naval Medicine, 1600–1830* (Amsterdam: Rodopi, 2007), 23–50.

Anderson, Richard, 'The diaspora of Sierra Leone's liberated Africans: Enlistment, forced migration, and "liberation" at Freetown, 1808–1863', *African Economic History* 41 (2013), 101–38.

Arnold, David, 'India's place in the tropical world, 1770–1930', *The Journal of Imperial and Commonwealth History* 26 (1998), 1–21.

Arnold, David, 'Race, place and bodily difference in early nineteenth-century India', *Historical Research* 77 (2004), 254–73.

Augustein, Hannah Franziska (ed.), *Race: the Origins of an Idea, 1760–1850* (Bristol: Thoemmes Press, 1996).

Beasley, Edward, 'Making races', *Victorian Review* 40 (2014), 48–52.

Beasley, Edward, *The Victorian Reinvention of Race* (New York: Routledge, 2010).

Beckett, Ian F. W., 'Manipulating the modern curse of armies: Wolseley, the press, and the Ashanti war, 1873–1874', in Stephen M. Miller (ed.), *Soldiers and Settlers in Africa, 1850–1918* (Brill: Leiden, 2009), 221–34.

Beckles, Hilary McD., 'A "riotous and unruly lot": Irish indentured servants and freemen in the English West Indies, 1644–1713', *William and Mary Quarterly* 47 (1990), 503–22.

Beckles, Hilary McD., 'An economic life of their own: Slaves as commodity producers and distributors in Barbados', *Slavery and Abolition* 21 (1991), 31–47.

Bennett, Melissa, 'Picturing the West India regiments: Race, empire, and photography c.1850–1914', unpublished PhD Dissertation, University of Warwick (2018).

Berlin, Ira, *Slaves without Masters: the Free Negro in the Antebellum South* (New York: Pantheon Books, 1974).

Blanco, R. L., 'The development of British military medicine, 1793–1814', *Military Affairs*, 38 (1974), 4–10.

Block, Sharon, *Colonial Complexions: Race and Bodies in Eighteenth Century America* (Philadelphia: University of Pennsylvania Press, 2018).

Bollettino, Maria Alessandra, '"Of equal or of more service": Black soldiers and the British empire in the mid-eighteenth-century Caribbean', *Slavery and Abolition* 38 (2017), 510–33.

Bond, Brian, *Victorian Military Campaigns* (London: Hutchinson, 1967).

Brace, C. Loring, 'The "ethnology" of Josiah Clark Nott', *Bulletin of the New York Academy of Medicine* 50 (1974), 509–28.

Brantlinger, Patrick, *Dark Vanishings: Discourse on the Extinction of Primitive Races, 1800–1930* (Ithaca: Cornell University Press, 2003).

Braude, Benjamin, 'The sons of Noah and the construction of ethnic and geographical identities in the medieval and early modern periods', *William and Mary Quarterly* 54 (1997), 103–42.

Breen, T. H. and Stephen Innes, *'Myne owne ground': Race and Freedom on Virginia's Eastern Shore, 1640–1676*, 2nd ed. (Oxford: Oxford University Press, 2005).

Bridenbaugh, Carl and Roberta Bridenbaugh, *No Peace Beyond the Line: the English in the Caribbean 1624–1690* (New York: Oxford University Press, 1972).

Brown, Christopher Leslie and Philip D. Morgan (eds.), *Arming Slaves from Classical Times to the Modern Age* (New Haven: Yale University Press, 2006).

Brown, B. Riccardo, *Until Darwin, Science, Human Variety and the Origins of Race* (London: Pickering and Chatto, 2010).

Brown, Spencer H., 'A tool of empire: the British medical establishment in Lagos, 1861–1905', *The International Journal of African Historical Studies* 37 (2004), 309–43.

Brown, Spencer H., 'British surgeons commissioned 1840–1909 with West Indian/West African service: a prosopographical evaluation', *Medical History* 37 (1993), 411–31.

Brown, Spencer H., 'Colonialism on the cheap: a tale of two English army surgeons in Lagos, Samuel Rowe and Frank Simpson, 1862–1882', *The International Journal of African Historical Studies* 27 (1994), 551–88.

Browne, Randy M., *Surviving Slavery in the British Caribbean* (Philadelphia: University of Pennsylvania Press, 2017).

Buckley, Roger N. (ed.), 'Brigadier-General Thomas Hislop's remarks on the establishment of the West India regiments – 1801', *Journal of the Society for Army Historical Research* 58 (1980), 209–22.

Buckley, Roger, *Slaves in Red Coats: the British West India Regiments, 1795–1815* (New Haven: Yale University Press, 1979).

Burnard, Trevor, *Mastery, Tyranny and Desire: Thomas Thistlewood and His Slaves in the Anglo-Jamaican World* (Chapel Hill: University of North Carolina Press, 2004).

Burnard, Trevor, 'Not a place for whites? Demographic failure and settlement in comparative perspective, 1655–1780', in Kathleen E. A. Monteith and Glen Richards (eds.), *Jamaica in Slavery and Freedom: History, Heritage and Culture* (Barbados: University of the West Indies Press, 2002), 73–88.

Burroughs, Peter, 'Crime and punishment in the British Army, 1815–1870', *English Historical Review* 100 (1985), 545–71.

Charters, Erica, 'Making bodies modern: Race, medicine and the colonial soldier in the mid-eighteenth century', *Patterns of Prejudice* 46 (2012), 214–31.

Chernin, Eli, 'Josiah Clark Nott, insects, and yellow fever', *Bulletin of the New York Academy of Medicine* 59 (1983), 790–802.

Churchill, Wendy D., 'Efficient, efficacious and humane responses to non-European bodies in British military medicine, 1780–1815', *The Journal of Imperial and Commonwealth History* 40 (2012), 137–58.

Cohn, Raymond L. and Richard A. Jensen, 'Mortality in the Atlantic slave trade', *The Journal of Interdisciplinary History* 13 (1982), 317–29.

Commissioned Officers in the Medical Service of the British Army, 1660–1960 (London: Wellcome Historical Medical Library, 1968).

Conway, Stephen, 'The mobilization of manpower for Britain's mid-eighteenth-century wars', *Historical Research* 77 (2004), 377–404.

Cooper, Elizabeth, 'Playing against empire', *Slavery and Abolition* 39 (2018), 540–57.

Cordingley, David, *Cochrane the Dauntless: the Life and Adventures of Admiral Thomas Cochrane, 1775–1860* (London: Bloomsbury, 2007).

Curran, Andrew, *The Anatomy of Blackness: Science and Slavery in an Age of Enlightenment* (Baltimore: John Hopkins University Press, 2011).

Curtin, Philip D., 'African health at home and abroad', *Social Science History* 10 (1986), 369–98.

Curtin, Philip D., 'The end of the "white man's grave"? Nineteenth-century mortality in west Africa', *The Journal of Interdisciplinary History* 21 (1990), 63–98.

Curtin, Philip D., *The Image of Africa: British Ideas and Action* (Madison: University of Wisconsin Press, 1964).

Dain, Bruce, *A Hideous Monster of the Mind: American Race Theory in the Early Republic* (Cambridge and London: Harvard University Press, 2002).

Delbourgo, James, *Collecting the World: the Life and Curiosity of Hans Sloane* (London: Penguin, 2017).

Desmond, Adrian and James Moore, *Darwin's Sacred Cause: Race, Slavery and the Quest for Human Origins* (London: Allen Lane, 2009).

Downs, W. G., 'Yellow fever and Josiah Clark Nott', *Bulletin of the New York Academy of Medicine* 50 (1974), 499–508.

Drescher, Seymour, 'The ending of the slave trade and the evolution of European scientific racism', *Social Science History* 14 (1990), 415–50.

Dunn, Richard S., *Sugar and slaves: the Rise of the Planter Class in the English West Indies, 1624–1713* (Chapel Hill: University of North Carolina Press, 1972).

Elkins, Stanley, *Slavery: a Problem in American Institutional and Intellectual Life* (Chicago: University of Chicago Press, 1959).

Eltis, David, *The Rise of African Slavery in the Americas* (Cambridge: Cambridge University Press, 2000).

Erickson, Paul, 'The anthropology of Josiah Clark Nott', *Kroeber Anthropological Society Papers* 65–66 (1986), 103–20.

Ericson, David F., *The Debate over Slavery: Antislavery and Proslavery Liberalism in Antebellum America* (New York: New York University Press, 2000).

Erikson, Emily, *Between Monopoly and Free Trade: the English East India Company, 1600–1757* (Princeton: Princeton University Press, 2014).

Fields, Barbara J., 'Ideology and race in American history', in J. Morgan Kousset and James M. McPherson (eds.), *Region, Race and Reconstruction: Essays in Honor of C. Vann Woodward* (New York: Oxford University Press, 1982), 143–77.

Foner, Eric, *Reconstruction: America's Unfinished Revolution, 1863–1877* (New York: Harper and Row, 1988).

Franklin, John Hope, *Reconstruction after the Civil War* (Chicago: University of Chicago Press, 1961).

Games, Alison, 'Migration', in David Armitage and Michael J. Braddick (eds.), *The British Atlantic World 1500–1800* (New York: Palgrave, 2002), 33–52.

Geggus, David, *Slavery, War and Revolution: the British Occupation of Saint Domingue, 1793–1798* (New York: Oxford University Press, 1982).

Geggus, David, 'The cost of Pitt's Caribbean campaigns, 1793–1798', *The Historical Journal* 26 (1983), 699–706.

Genovese, Eugene, *Roll, Jordan, Roll: the World the Slaves Made* (New York: Pantheon Books, 1974).

Gorges, Howard, *The Great War in West Africa* (London: Naval and Military Press, 2004).

Gould, Stephen Jay, *The Mismeasure of Man* (New York: Norton, 1996).

Greene, John C., 'Darwin as a social evolutionist', *Journal of the History of Biology* 10 (1977), 1–27.

Gross, Ariela J., 'Litigating whiteness: Trials of racial determination in the nineteenth-century South', *The Yale Law Journal* 108 (1998), 109–88.

Guerra, F., 'The influence of disease on race, logistics and colonization in the Antilles', *Journal of Tropical Medicine and Hygiene* 49 (1966), 23–35.

Hall, Neville, 'Slaves use of their "free time" in the Danish Virgin islands in the later eighteenth and early nineteenth century', *Journal of Caribbean History* 13 (1980), 21–43.

Haller, John S., *Outcasts from Evolution: Scientific Attitudes of Racial Inferiority, 1859–1900* (Chicago: University of Illinois Press, 1971).

Harrison, Mark, *Climates and Constitutions: Health, Race, Environment and British Imperialism in India, 1600–1850* (Oxford: Oxford University Press, 1999).

Harrison, Mark, *Medicine in an Age of Commerce and Empire: Britain and Its Tropical Colonies, 1660–1830* (Oxford: Oxford University Press, 2010).

Henze, Brent, 'Scientific definition in rhetorical formations: Race as "permanent variety" in James Cowles Prichard's ethnology', *Rhetoric Review* 23 (2004), 311–31.

Heuman, Gad J., *Between Black and White: Race, Politics, and the Free Coloreds in Jamaica, 1792–1865* (Westport: Greenwood Press, 1981).

Heuman, Gad J., *The Caribbean: a Brief History*, 2nd ed. (London: Bloomsbury, 2014).

Higman, Barry W., *Slave Populations of the British Caribbean 1807–1834* (Kingston, Jamaica: University of the West Indies Press, 1995).

Hogarth, Rana A., *Medicalizing Blackness: Making Racial Difference in the Atlantic World, 1780–1840* (Chapel Hill: University of North Carolina Press, 2017).

Horsman, Reginald, *Josiah Nott of Mobile: Southerner, Physician, and Racial Theorist* (Baton Rouge: Louisiana State University Press, 1987).

Howe, Glenford D., *Race, War and Nationalism: a Social History of West Indians in the First World War* (Oxford: James Currey, 2002).

Johnson, Katherine, 'The constitution of empire: Place and bodily health in the eighteenth-century Atlantic', *Atlantic Studies* 10 (2013), 443–66.

Jones, Randolph, 'The Bourbon Regiment and the Barbados slave revolt of 1816', *Journal of the Society for Army Historical Research* 78 (2000), 3–10.

Jordan, Winthrop, *The White Man's Burden: Historical Origins of Racism in the United States* (New York: Oxford University Press, 1974).

Jordan, Winthrop, *White over Black: American Attitudes Towards the Negro* (Chapel Hill: University of North Carolina Press, 1968).

Joseph, Michael, 'Military officers, tropical medicine, and racial thought in the formation of the West India regiments, 1793–1802', *Journal of the History of Medicine*, 72 (2017), 142–65.

Keel, Terence D., 'Religion, polygenism and the early science of human origins', *History of the Human Sciences* 26 (2013), 3–32.

Kelly, Catherine, *War and the Militarization of British Army Medicine, 1793–1830* (London: Pickering and Chatto, 2011).

Kidd, Colin, *The Forging of Races: Race and Scripture in the Protestant Atlantic World, 1600–2000* (Cambridge: Cambridge University Press, 2006).

King, Stewart, *Blue Coat or Powdered Wig: Free People of Color in Pre-Revolutionary Saint Domingue* (Athens: University of Georgia Press, 2001).

Kiple, Kenneth F. and Virginia H. Kiple, 'Black yellow fever immunities, innate and acquired, as revealed in the American South', *Social Science History* 1 (1977), 419–36.

Klein, Herbert S. and Stanley L. Engerman, 'Long-term trends in African mortality in the transatlantic slave trade', *Slavery and Abolition* 18 (1997), 36–48.

Kupperman, Karen Ordahl, 'Fear of hot climates in the Anglo-American colonial experience', *William and Mary Quarterly* 41 (1984), 213–40.

Lambert, David, '"[A] mere cloak for their proud contempt and antipathy towards the African race": Imagining Britain's West India regiments in the Caribbean, 1795–1838', *Journal of Imperial and Commonwealth History* 46 (2018), 627–50.

Livingstone, David N., *Adam's Ancestors: Race, Religion and the Politics of Human Origins* (Baltimore: Johns Hopkins University Press, 2008).

Livingstone, David N., 'Human acclimatization: Perspectives on a contested field of inquiry in science, medicine, and geography', *History of Science* 25 (1987), 359–94.

Lorimer, Douglas A., *Colour, Class and the Victorians: English Attitudes to the Negro in the Mid-Nineteenth Century* (Leicester: Leicester University Press, 1978).

Luse, Christopher A., 'Slavery's champions stood at odds: Polygenesis and the defense of slavery', *Civil War History* 53 (2007), 379–412.

McNeill, J. R., *Mosquito Empires: Ecology and War in the Greater Caribbean, 1620–1914* (Cambridge: Cambridge University Press, 2010).

Marshall, Woodville K., 'Provision ground and plantation labor in four Windward Islands: Competition for resources during slavery', *Slavery and Abolition* 21 (1991), 48–67.

Michael, C., A. Johansson, Neysarí Arana-Vizcarrondo, Brad J. Biggerstaff, and J. Erin Staples, 'Incubation periods of yellow fever virus', *American Journal of Tropical Medicine* 83 (2010), 183–8.

Mintz, Sidney W. and Douglas Hall, *The Origins of the Jamaican Internal Marketing System* (New Haven: Yale University Press, 1970).

Oakes, James, '"Whom have I oppressed?" The pursuit of happiness and the happy slave', in James Horn et al. (eds.), *The Revolution of 1800: Democracy, Race and the New Republic* (Charlottesville: University of Virginia Press, 2002), 220–39.

Orr, G. M., 'The origin of the West India regiment', *Journal of the Royal United Service Institution* 72 (1927), 129–30.

Paugh, Katherine, 'Yaws, syphilis, sexuality, and the circulation of medical knowledge in the British Caribbean and the Atlantic world', *Bulletin of the History of Medicine* 88 (2014), 225–52.

Pernick, Martin S., *A Calculus of Suffering: Pain, Professionalism, and Anesthesia in Nineteenth-Century America* (New York: Columbia University Press, 1985).

Phillips, Christopher, *Freedom's Port: the African American Community of Baltimore, 1790–1860* (Urbana: University of Illinois Press, 1997).

Polk, William M., 'Josiah C. Nott', *American Journal of Obstetrics* 67 (1913), 957.

Porter, Theodore M., *The Rise of Statistical Thinking* (Princeton: Princeton University Press, 1986).

Powell, J. H., *Bring Out Your Dead: the Great Plague of Yellow Fever in Philadelphia, in 1793* (Philadelphia: University of Pennsylvania Press, 1949).

Rankin, John, *Healing the African Body: British Medicine in West Africa, 1800–1860* (Columbia, Missouri, University of Missouri Press, 2015).

Richards, Evelleen, 'The "moral anatomy" of Robert Knox: the interplay between biological and social thought in Victorian scientific naturalism', *Journal of the History of Biology* 22 (1989), 373–436.

Russett, Cynthia Eagle, *Darwin in America: the Intellectual Response, 1865–1912* (San Francisco: W. H. Freeman, 1976).

Savitt, Todd L., *Medicine and Slavery: the Diseases and Healthcare of Blacks in Antebellum Virginia* (Urbana and Chicago: University of Illinois Press, 1981).

Scanlan, Padraic X., *Freedom's Debtors: British Antislavery in Sierra Leone in the Age of Revolution* (New Haven: Yale University Press, 2017).

Schiebinger, Londa, *Secret Cures of Slaves: People, Plants and Medicine and the Eighteenth-Century Atlantic World* (Stanford: Stanford University Press, 2017).

Schneider, Elena A., *The Occupation of Havana: War, Trade, and Slavery in the Atlantic World* (Chapel Hill: University of North Carolina Press, 2018).

Sellick, Gary, 'Black skin, red coats: the Carolina corps and nationalism in the revolutionary British Caribbean', *Slavery and Abolition* 39 (2018), 459–78.

Seth, Suman, *Difference and Disease: Medicine, Race and the Eighteenth-Century British Empire* (Cambridge: Cambridge University Press, 2018).

Sheridan, Richard B., *Doctors and Slaves: a Medical and Demographic History of Slavery in the British West Indies, 1680–1834* (Cambridge: Cambridge University Press, 1985).

Sheridan, Richard B., 'The Guinea surgeons on the middle passage: the provision of medical services in the British slave trade', *The International Journal of African Historical Studies* 14 (1981), 601–25.

Sheridan, Richard B., 'Sir William Young (1749–1815): Planter and politician, with special reference to slavery in the British West Indies', *Journal of Caribbean History* 33 (1999), 1–26.

Smith, Billy G., *Ship of Death: a Voyage That Changed the Atlantic World* (New Haven: Yale University Press, 2013).

Smith, Billy G. and J. Worth Estes, *"A Melancholy Scene of Devastation": the Public Response to the 1793 Philadelphia Yellow Fever Epidemic* (Philadelphia: Science History Publications, 1997).

Smith, John David (ed.), *Black Soldiers in Blue: African American Troops in the Civil War Era* (Chapel Hill: University of North Carolina Press, 2002).

Smith, Mark M., *How Race Is Made: Slavery, Segregation and the Senses* (Chapel Hill: University of North Carolina Press, 2006).

Smith, Richard, *Jamaican Volunteers in the First World War: Race, Masculinity and the Development of National Consciousness* (Manchester: Manchester University Press, 2004).

Spielman, Andrew and Michael D'Antonio, *Mosquito: a Natural History of Our Most Persistent and Deadly Foe* (New York: Hyperion, 2001).

Stepan, Nancy, *Idea of Race in Science* (London: Macmillan, 1982).

Steppler, G. A., 'British military law, discipline, and the conduct of regimental courts martial in the later eighteenth century', *The English Historical Review* 102 (1987), 859–86.

Sweet, James H., 'The Iberian roots of American racist thought', *William and Mary Quarterly* 54 (1997), 143–66.

Tinker, Tink and Mark Freeland, 'Thief, slave trader, murderer: Christopher Columbus and Caribbean population decline', *Wicazo sa Review* 23 (2008), 25–50.

Tyson, George F., 'The Carolina Black corps: Legacy of revolution (1782–1798)', *Revista/Review Interamericana* 5 (1975/6), 661–3.

Ukpabi, Samson C., 'Military recruitment and social mobility in nineteenth century British west Africa', *Journal of African Studies* 2 (1975), 87–107.

Vandervort, Bruce, *Wars of Imperial Conquest in Africa, 1830–1914* (Bloomington: Indiana University Press, 1998).

Vetch, R. H., *Life of Lieutenant-General the Hon. Sir Andrew Clarke* (London: J. Murray, 1905).

Voelz, Peter M., *Slave and Soldier: the Military Impact of Blacks in the Colonial Americas* (New York: London: Garland, 1993).

Walvin, James, *England, Slaves and Freedom, 1776–1838* (London: Macmillan, 1986).

Walvin, James, *Questioning Slavery* (London: Routledge, 1996).

Wheeler, Roxann, *The Complexion of Race: Categories of Difference in Eighteenth-Century British Culture* (Philadelphia: University of Pennsylvania Press, 2000).

Williamson, Joel, *New People: Miscegenation and Mulattoes in the United States.* (New York: Free Press, 1980).

Willoughby, Christopher D. E., 'Running away from drapetomania: Samuel A. Cartwright, medicine, and race in the antebellum South', *Journal of Southern History* 84 (2018), 579–614.

Wills, Christopher, *Yellow Fever – Black Goddess: the Coevolution of People and Plagues* (Reading, PA: Addison-Wesley, 1996).

Wood, Betty, *The Origins of American Slavery: Freedom and Bondage in the English Colonies* (London: Hill and Wang, 1998).

Young, Jeffrey Robert (ed.), *Proslavery and Sectional Thought in the Early South, 1740–1829* (Columbia: University of South Carolina Press, 2006).

Index